# ESSENTIALS OF
# PHARMACOLOGY
## FOR NURSING PRACTICE

# ESSENTIALS OF PHARMACOLOGY
## FOR NURSING PRACTICE

ALISON BUCKLEY
JULIA ROBINSON
MARK MAGAS

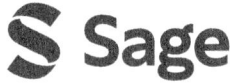

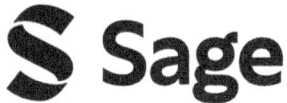

1 Oliver's Yard
55 City Road
London EC1Y 1SP

2455 Teller Road
Thousand Oaks
California 91320

Unit No 323-333, Third Floor, F-Block
International Trade Tower
Nehru Place, New Delhi – 110 019

8 Marina View Suite 43-053
Asia Square Tower 1
Singapore 018960

Editor: Laura Walmsley
Assistant editor: Sahar Jamfar
Production editor: Martin Fox
Copyeditor: William Baginsky
Proofreader: Tom Bedford
Marketing manager: Ruslana Khatagova
Cover design: Sheila Tong
Typeset by: C&M Digitals (P) Ltd, Chennai, India
Printed in the UK

© Alison Buckley, Julia Robinson and Mark Magas 2025

Apart from any fair dealing for the purposes of research, private study, or criticism or review, as permitted under the Copyright, Designs and Patents Act, 1988, this publication may not be reproduced, stored or transmitted in any form, or by any means, without the prior permission in writing of the publisher, or in the case of reprographic reproduction, in accordance with the terms of licences issued by the Copyright Licensing Agency. Enquiries concerning reproduction outside those terms should be sent to the publisher.

Library of Congress Control Number: 2024942891

**British Library Cataloguing in Publication data**

A catalogue record for this book is available from the British Library

ISBN 978-1-5296-0903-5
ISBN 978-1-5296-0902-8 (pbk)

# CONTENTS

*About the authors*     vii
*Foreword*     ix
*Preface*     xi

1. Introducing Pharmacology: Scientific Principles and Concepts     1
2. Routes of Drug Administration and Drug Absorption     29
3. Drug Distribution     63
4. Drug Metabolism     79
5. Drug Excretion     101
6. Principles of Pharmacodynamics     113
7. Case Studies: Applying Principles to Nursing Practice     141

*Bibliography*     165
*Glossary*     167
*Index*     175

# ABOUT THE AUTHORS

**Alison Buckley**, a Doctor of Philosophy in Nursing, is a Senior Lecturer in Nursing at the University of Cumbria. She has a long history of leading and developing nursing curricula, with particular academic and professional interests in ethics, law, professional practice, pathophysiology, pharmacology, medicine and neurocritical care. Her research interests lie in the lived experience of disordered consciousness secondary to acquired brain injury, applied phenomenology and narrative inquiry. She currently takes a lead role in pre-registration nursing education and remains a Registered Nurse with the Nursing and Midwifery Council (UK).

**Julia Robinson** is a Senior Lecturer in Children's Nursing at the University of Central Lancashire. Julia teaches pharmacology to undergraduate nursing students as part of their pre-registration curriculum. Julia is a Non-Medical Prescriber and, along with Alison Buckley, she edited *Preparation for Prescribing: Medicine Management & Applied Pharmacology*, a digital resource produced by the Health & Education Cooperative which has been adopted by several universities across the UK. She is a Fellow of the Higher Education Academy (FHEA).

**Mark Magas** is a Senior Lecturer in Pharmacology at the University of Cumbria and Subject Lead for Pharmacology and Prescribing at the Pears Cumbria School of Medicine. Mark teaches pharmacology to undergraduate biomedical sciences students, and other healthcare professionals. He has had many years of experience teaching on postgraduate non-medical prescribing programmes in the past and is currently working with the postgraduate medical school on pharmacology and prescribing. Mark is a Pharmacist, registered with the GPhC and a Fellow of the Institute of Biomedical Science.

# FOREWORD

Nursing, as a profession, continues to be a central and pivotal part of delivering evidence-based patient-centred care. Over the years, the role of the nurse continues to grow in its scope, leading to a range of career paths for nurses: from working in a range of practice settings to further developing knowledge and skills such as advanced clinical practitioners, specialist community nurses or mental health nurses with a range of psychosocial therapeutic skills, to name just a few. These changes over the years have continued to emphasise the need for the nursing profession to ensure they are equipped with the right knowledge, the right skills and the ability to ensure evidence-based practice in a range of settings and across *all* fields of nursing.

Having been a registered nurse since 1985, I have been able to witness the profession of nursing and, as an academic, I have been able to develop curricula that supports the ever-changing scope of professional practice required by nurses, all of which requires a greater understanding of science-based knowledge, developing clinical skills, communication skills and, of course, how these work together in their application to patient-centred care in all fields of nursing. Currently, in 2025 the evolution of the nursing profession continues against a backdrop of nursing workforce shortages (at a global level as well as across the UK) and fewer members of the population finding nursing as an attractive career choice as perhaps it once was.

In 2018, the Nursing and Midwifery Council (NMC) published their *Future Nurse Standards of Proficiency for Registered Nurses* which placed a greater emphasis on the role and scope of the nursing profession, a much-needed change in my view. Within those standards, pharmacology and its application to nursing practice is identified as a key requirement of the future nurse, which makes the timing and focus of this book an essential read for all nursing students, as well registered nurses who are further developing their knowledge and careers. Within my own career, I have always found pharmacology and its application to practice a difficult and challenging area of learning, which I regarded as overly complex and perhaps a bit too theoretical. If only this book had been written then!

At its heart, *Essentials of Pharmacology for Nursing Practice* assumes no previous knowledge, which given the many routes into the nursing profession is an encouraging approach as it takes the reader on a journey of understanding, learning and clinical practice. Not only does it provide an evidence-based approach to understanding pharmacological principles, but it also provides the reader with a strong focus on physiological concepts and their application of this knowledge to real life clinical scenarios. This book has been purposefully designed to provide the reader with a clear understanding of how pharmacological principles can be applied in clinical practice and in a range of settings. Threaded throughout the chapters of this book are clinical examples which I believe readers will relate to as they reflect real life scenarios. Helpfully, this book doesn't aim to just provide you with facts, rather it carefully takes you on a journey of understanding, relating principles, physiology, clinical practice and your role.

However, it is my view that this book will do more than you expect. Whilst it will give you essential knowledge it will also provide you with a confidence to practise the profession of nursing and apply your new knowledge of pharmacology to the care of individuals. I believe it will support your development to practise safely and underpin your knowledge with evidence, all of which should provide you, the reader, with confidence in practice and for the future.

The *Future Nurse Standards*, in my view, don't just equip you for the here and now, they provide a platform for you to further develop your career from student nurse to registered nurse in a context of a continually evolving and changing profession. Pharmacology and its application to safe patient care isn't just important for you whilst you are student or a new learner, it's an important pillar of professional practice for the future of your career.

Finally, I would encourage you, as the reader, to take the time to reflect on your new learning as you read and work through each chapter. This is not a book that you just read to learn new facts, this is a book that will support your learning, guide you in the application of your new learning and support you to apply your new learning to patient-centred care, which in my view, is a successful aspect of the authors' approach to you, the reader.

Professor Brian Webster-Henderson OBE

Deputy Vice Chancellor, University of Cumbria

Professor of Nursing

Fellow of the Queen's Nursing Institute

# PREFACE

This book is intended to introduce the reader to the principles and practice of pharmacology, with a particular focus on pharmacokinetics and pharmacodynamics as applied to clinical practice.

The British National Formulary (BNF), Electronic Medicines Compendium (EMC), National Institute for Health and Care Excellence (NICE) and regulatory bodies (e.g. the Medicines and Healthcare products Regulatory Agency (MHRA)) provide evidence-based information relating to medicine optimisation, efficacy, safety and regulation. Please be encouraged to access these resources alongside this text. The regulation and practice of medicine prescribing, monitoring and post-marketing surveillance are dynamic and ongoing processes, and subject to review and development. It is therefore important to keep abreast of any changes to optimise your understanding of the clinical application of pharmacology and medicine therapeutics.

The textbook comprises seven chapters. Chapter 1 introduces the reader to key scientific principles relevant to the principles and practice of pharmacology. Chapters 2 to 5 are organised according to the pharmacokinetics principles: Absorption, Distribution, Metabolism and Excretion. Each chapter will define key concepts related to pharmacokinetics, informed by relevant anatomy and physiology, and provide working examples of drugs that are prescribed. Chapter 6 addresses the principles of pharmacodynamics. The final chapter, Chapter 7, presents case studies to enable you to apply the pharmacological principles explained throughout the preceding chapters and considers aspects of clinical decision making, to inform safe and therapeutic practice in medicine management.

# INTRODUCING PHARMACOLOGY 1
## SCIENTIFIC PRINCIPLES AND CONCEPTS

---
### LEARNING OUTCOMES
---

By the end of this chapter, you should be able to:

1. Define and explain key scientific and physiological concepts which inform the principles and practice of pharmacokinetics and pharmacodynamics
2. Introduce the study of pharmacology in the context of safe and therapeutic medicine management
3. Explain drug **nomenclature**

## INTRODUCTION

The aim of Chapter 1 is to introduce a range of scientific principles and concepts which will provide a background to the theoretical underpinnings of **pharmacology** presented in this book. Key definitions and concepts will be introduced to help inform your understanding of fundamental physiological and biochemical pathways. Essential bioscience will be explored and its relevance to the application and understanding of pharmacological principles explained.

The human body is fundamentally a collection of cellular processes which collectively inform physiological functioning. In the development and progression of disease – *dis-ease* – there are fundamental derangements in these physiological processes which result in cellular, organ and system dysfunction.

To appreciate the principles of pharmacology (i.e. the mode of action of drugs and how the human body affects drug movement from the site of administration to excretion) it is necessary to review several fundamental biochemical and physiological principles.

It is anticipated that this chapter will need to be revisited as concepts described will inform several pharmacological concepts discussed throughout the following chapters.

Pharmacology is an overarching term which involves the understanding of a drug's mode of action on the body and the way in which the body affects drug movement from the point of drug administration through to drug excretion. An understanding and appreciation of these fundamental concepts ensures that the desired therapeutic response is realised, with the aim of optimising treatment outcomes and ensuring the safe and therapeutic use of medicines.

There are several branches of pharmacology, including **pharmacokinetics** and **pharmacodynamics**, both summarised below.

*Pharmacokinetics* is the study of drug movement through the body and how the body handles the drug. The pharmacokinetic stages are summarised as ADME:

A: **Absorption**

D: **Distribution**

M: **Metabolism**

E: **Excretion** or Elimination

*Pharmacodynamics* is the study of the mode of action of the drug: how the drug acts to prevent or manage disease and the related signs and symptoms.

## DRUG NOMENCLATURE

To explain key pharmacological concepts, examples of drugs will be given throughout the chapters. It is therefore important that the International Nonproprietary Names (INN) and/or British Approved Names (BAN) are used. This is also referred to as the *generic* name. A capital letter is not used, and the name begins in lower case. The stem or affix will indicate the group to which the drug belongs (Table 1.1).

The *trademark name* or *brand name* which is given by the pharmaceutical company begins with a capital letter (note that brand name availability may be subject to change).

There are several physiological concepts and principles which need to be understood so that you can apply these to the study of the principles and practice of pharmacology.

An understanding of human physiology and anatomy also helps to understand why drugs are prescribed either as preventative measures or in the management of disease and/or the clinical manifestations seen.

---

### PAUSE AND REFLECT 1.1

Think of several drugs that you are familiar with and identify the International Nonproprietary Name and/or British Approved Name and trademark/brand name for each one.

**Table 1.1** Drug actions and names

| 'stem' or 'affix' | Drug action | International Nonproprietary Name and/or British Approved Name | Trademark or brand name |
| --- | --- | --- | --- |
| -olol | Beta-blockers to manage hypertension | atenolol | Tenormin (AstraZeneca UK Ltd) |
| -profen | Non-steroidal anti-inflammatory drugs | ibuprofen | Brufen (Mylan Ltd) |
|  |  |  | Nurofen (Reckitt-Benckiser Healthcare UK Ltd) |
|  |  |  | Ibucalm (Aspar Pharmaceuticals Ltd) |
|  |  | ketoprofen | Larafen CR (Ennogen Pharma Ltd) |
|  |  |  | Oruvail (Sanofi UK) |
| -pril | Angiotensin-converting enzyme (ACE) inhibitors to manage hypertension | enalapril | Innovace (Merck Sharp & Dohme Ltd) |
|  |  | captopril | Capoten (Bristol-Myers Squibb Pharmaceuticals Ltd) |
|  |  | lisinopril | Zestril (AstraZeneca UK Ltd) |
| -cillin | Penicillin-derived antibacterials | amoxicillin | Amoxil (GlaxoSmithKline UK Ltd) |

## PHYSIOLOGICAL CONCEPTS AND PRINCIPLES

### Homeostasis

**Homeostasis** is a biological concept whereby organisms and **cells** maintain an internal, regulated environment to promote stability and control. The maintenance of this internal control ensures that physiological functioning is optimised despite changes to the external environment. Homeostatic processes control, for example, the regulation of body temperature (thermoregulation), water balance (osmoregulation), electrolyte balance (e.g. sodium, potassium and calcium levels), the **pH** of the blood and blood glucose levels. Without these homeostatic mechanisms there would be significant derangements in cell functioning leading to organ and system dysfunction.

Without exception, all body systems employ homeostatic mechanisms to ensure internal control (Figure 1.1).

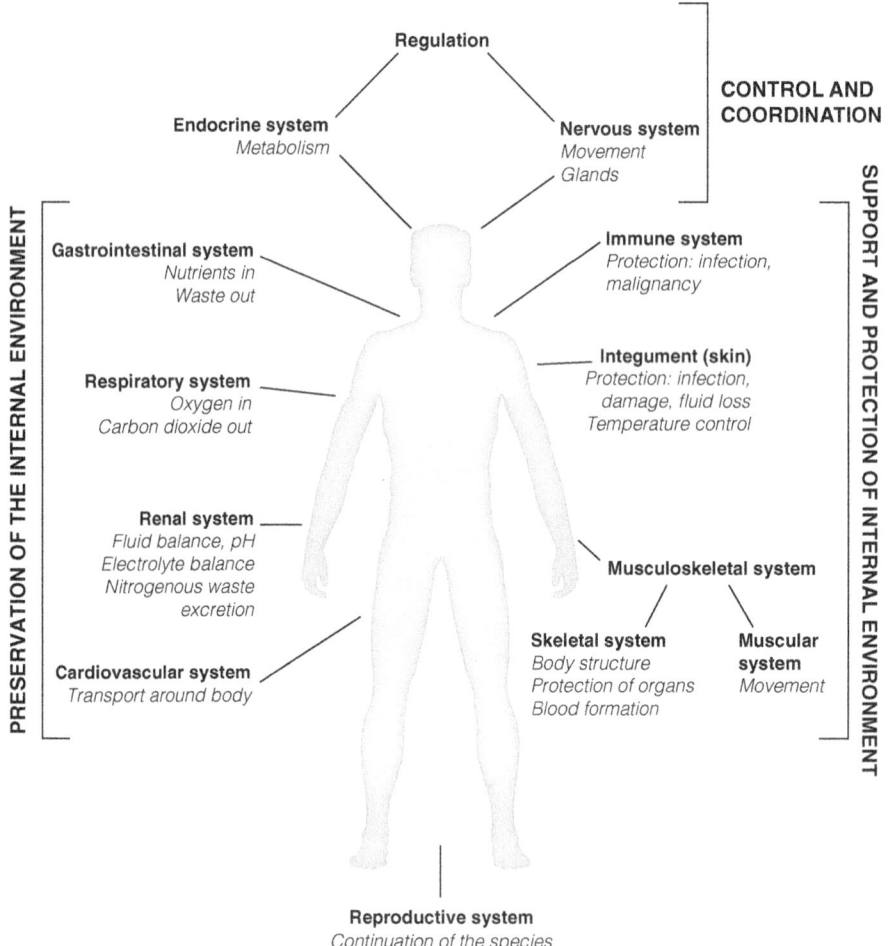

**Figure 1.1** The Internal Environment

Homeostatic control mechanisms generally include three independent but related elements:

1. A **detector** or **receptor** which monitors internal control and detects the derangement
2. A *control centre*
3. An **effector** or target site which is acted upon to bring about the change

Let's explore these three elements further through the examples of the homeostatic control of respiration and of blood pressure.

## The Homeostatic Control of Respiration

*The detectors/receptors*: The oxygen, carbon dioxide levels and pH of the blood are continually monitored by central and peripheral **chemoreceptors**. These chemoreceptors will detect derangements in the blood chemistry. If respiration is inadequate, then there will be lower oxygen levels and higher carbon dioxide levels in the arterial blood, with the latter resulting in an increase in $H^+$ (hydrogen ions) lowering the blood's pH. Central chemoreceptors situated in the medulla oblongata of the brainstem detect a rise in $H^+$ (hydrogen ions) with peripheral chemoreceptors detecting changes in arterial oxygenation. The chemoreceptors will send this information to the respiratory control centres found in the brainstem.

The respiratory control centres receive information from the chemoreceptors about the biochemistry of the arterial blood. There are several control centres in the brainstem:

- Medulla oblongata: The 'medullary rhythmicity' centre controls the inspiratory and expiratory phases of breathing.
- Pons varolii: The apneustic and pneumotaxic centres influence the inspiratory volume and the respiratory rate.

Collectively, these control centres will alter the rate, depth and rhythm of breathing through neural control.

The **effector organs** involve the structures of breathing (e.g. the intercostal muscles and the diaphragm) to effect changes to the rate, depth and rhythm of breathing to improve blood oxygenation and the exhalation of carbon dioxide.

## The Homeostatic Control of Blood Pressure

Another example of a homeostatic process is the control of systemic blood pressure (see Figure 1.2). Several neural and endocrine responses are activated when the systemic blood pressure is low. Baroreceptors located in the carotid sinus and the wall of the ascending aorta *detect* low pressure and send a neural message to the cardiovascular and vasomotor centres (control centres) in the medulla oblongata which in turn activate the sympathetic nervous system to increase cardiac output and cause peripheral vasoconstriction (*effectors*). These combined effector responses result in an increase in the systemic blood pressure. In addition, the renin-angiotensin-aldosterone pathway is activated along with the release of catecholamines, epinephrine and norepinephrine which collectively result in an increase in blood pressure.

Whilst there are many other examples of homeostatic processes in the body, it is important to understand these normal physiological mechanisms to better understand how derangements can result in disease and the nature of the pathophysiological change seen.

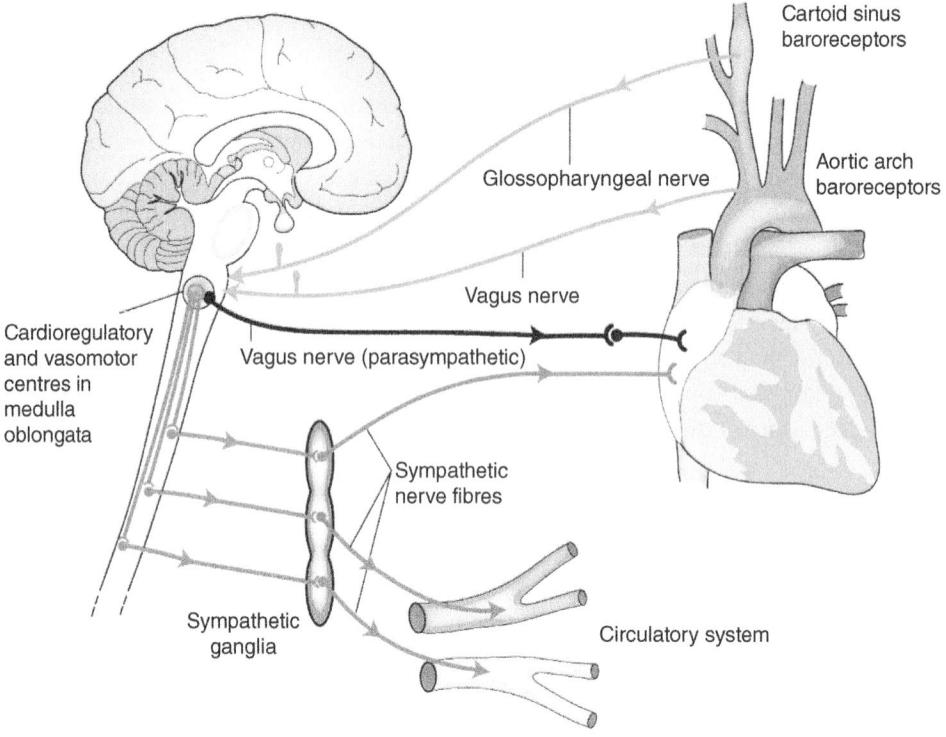

**Figure 1.2** Baroreceptor response

---

### PAUSE AND REFLECT 1.2

Consider another homeostatic mechanism within the body and identify the detector(s), control centre(s) and effector(s).

---

Drugs may be prescribed to manage the effects of homeostatic derangements and support the physiological parameters to return to acceptable levels.

## Atoms, Elements, Compounds and Molecules

Drugs are **molecules** and/or **compounds** which are made up of **atoms** and elements. It is therefore important to understand them in the context of drug development and their use as therapeutic agents.

### Atoms

Atoms are the principal building blocks of matter. Elements are formed from atoms and the atoms are the smallest part into which an element can be split. Elements, in turn, make up all substances in the universe.

## Elements

In chemistry, an element is a type of matter that consists of only one type of atom, and these are the basic building blocks of all chemical compounds, including the most complicated proteins and other macromolecules found in the human body. Most elements are found combined with others in the human body as compounds or as ions.

Of the 118 known elements, only some are found in the human body in great proportion, for example carbon, hydrogen, oxygen and nitrogen. These elements make up the proteins, carbohydrates and lipids that we are comprised of, whilst others are found in smaller proportions, such as sodium and calcium. Both elements have many functions. Sodium, for example, is involved in fluid balance, blood pressure regulation and nerve conduction, whilst calcium gives bones a solid structure and is involved in muscle contraction. Trace elements include iron, the most abundant trace element, necessary for oxygen transport, and cobalt, a component of vitamin B12, which is important for red blood cell formation. Although cobalt is present in small quantities, it is included in the hydroxocobalamin injection (see Table 1.2).

**Table 1.2** Common elements

| Element and symbol | Use in the human body | Found in |
|---|---|---|
| Iron (Fe) | Essential for oxygen transport in haemoglobin and electron transport in cellular respiration | Red meat, poultry, fish, beans and fortified cereals |
| Zinc (Zn) | Involved in enzyme function, immune system support and wound healing | Meat, dairy products, nuts and legumes |
| Copper (Cu) | Important for the formation of red blood cells and maintenance of connective tissues | Organ meats, seafood, nuts, seeds and whole grains |
| Iodine (I) | Essential for thyroid hormone synthesis, which regulates metabolism | Seafood, iodised salt, dairy products and some vegetables |
| Manganese (Mn) | Involved in bone formation, blood clotting and reducing oxidative stress | Nuts, seeds, whole grains and green leafy vegetables |
| Selenium (Se) | Acts as an antioxidant, supports the immune system and is involved in thyroid function | Seafood, meat, grains and Brazil nuts |
| Fluoride (F) | Promotes dental health by preventing tooth decay | Fluoridated water, tea and seafood |
| Chromium (Cr) | Enhances the action of insulin and helps regulate blood sugar | Broccoli, whole grains, meat and nuts |
| Molybdenum (Mo) | Participates in enzyme reactions, especially those involved in amino acid metabolism | Legumes, grains, nuts and leafy vegetables |
| Cobalt (Co) | A component of vitamin B12, which is essential for red blood cell formation | Fish, nuts and green leafy vegetables |

## Compounds

A compound is formed through the chemical bonding of two or more different chemical elements. Depending on how electrons are shared or passed between the atoms, these bonds can be either covalent or ionic. The characteristics of compounds are distinct from those of their component parts.

In pharmacology and physiology, it is important to have an appreciation of chemical formulae which represent compounds as they indicate the types and numbers of atoms present. For example, water is a compound with the chemical formula ($H_2O$), carbon dioxide ($CO_2$) and glucose ($C_6H_{12}O_6$). These are examples of compounds and their formulae. Ionic compounds involve the transfer of electrons, which have a negative charge, leading to the formation of positive and negative ions such as $Na^+$, $K^+$, $Ca^{2+}$ and $Cl^-$. The number indicates the number of electrons that have transferred (no number means '1') and the charge, positive '+' or negative '−' indicates whether the atoms have lost electrons and become more positive ('+') or gained them and become more negative ('−').

The other option in the human body is for a compound to be covalent. Covalency involves the sharing of electrons between atoms which can be very simple molecules, such as oxygen ($O_2$) or water ($H_2O$), or more complicated molecules such as phenylalanine ($C_9H_{11}NO_2$). We tend to represent things by their molecular formula only when they are relatively small molecules because for larger molecules, e.g. haemoglobin, the chemical formula becomes meaningless in medicine as it is difficult to imagine what that would look like when written as $C_{34}H_{33}FeN_4O_4$. The number in subscript indicates the number of atoms of that element in the compound.

## Molecules Versus Compounds

In the practice of medicine, the word 'molecule' is often used for drugs, as in 'drug molecules'.

However, strictly speaking, there is a difference between a molecule and a compound. Molecules are formed when atoms bond together. These atoms could be the same elements *or* from different elements, whereas a compound is always made up of bonding involving atoms of two or more different elements. Therefore, compounds always contain more than one type of element in a fixed ratio. So, all compounds are molecules but not all molecules are compounds. Most drugs are compounds but there is nothing wrong with calling them molecules as this catch-all term is always going to be correct.

For example, iodine ($I_2$) and oxygen ($O_2$) are only ever going to be described as molecules by chemists because they contain more than one atom. But molecules may also contain more than one type of atom as well. So, glucose ($C_6H_{12}O_6$) and common salt (NaCl) are molecules but are also compounds because compounds *must* have more than one element.

It can be confusing as terminology can be used interchangeably. For example, most people would say oxygen molecules and be fine with that, and this is correct. Conversely 'oxygen compound' would be wrong but we never hear people saying this anyway. However, water is a molecule but also a compound by the definition, so saying, 'the compound, water' would be correct, but no one ever would say this; it sounds wrong. We'd all stick to saying water molecules!

In summary, for drugs it is acceptable to say 'molecules' and no one reading or listening to you will think twice about it.

## Acids, Bases (Alkali) and the pH Scale

Many people have a basic understanding of what is meant by an **acid** or an alkali. So, before learning more about these chemical concepts, it is important to appreciate how they relate to pharmacology and physiology. In physiology, the pH of our body plays a significant role in **enzyme** activity, for example the enzymes in the small intestine work best in an alkaline pH whereas those in the stomach work optimally in an acidic environment. On a wider scale, certain diseases can alter the pH of bodily fluids either locally or throughout the body. For example, respiratory acidosis, which is an increase of acidity in the blood (decreased pH), typically results from lack of removal of carbon dioxide from the blood. The carbon dioxide dissolves to a greater extent in the blood, forming an acid. Therefore, monitoring pH changes can aid in the diagnosis and management of conditions such as acid–**base** imbalances, respiratory or metabolic disorders.

With respect to the study of pharmacology, the pH of the gastrointestinal (GI) tract can affect the solubility of drugs. Some drugs absorb in acidic environments (e.g. the stomach) while others are absorbed in more alkaline environments (e.g. the small intestine, although in practice the large surface area of the small intestine trumps these pH differences in terms of drug absorption). As another example, the ionisation state of a drug is pH dependent. This affects a drug's ability to cross cell membranes and distribute within the body. For example, a relatively small drug molecule that is largely ionised at body pH would not cross cell membranes easily and therefore would probably not get to its target site of action. Alternatively, a small uncharged molecule would be able to pass through the mainly lipid cell membranes more easily. Another example is local **anaesthetics**. They are often weak bases that work better in acidic environments. Adjusting the pH of the formulation to be slightly acidic can enhance their **efficacy**.

So, what are acids and bases, and what does pH mean? The best way to begin is to explain the derivation of pH and the pH scale. The pH quantifies how acidic, or not, something is. The pH scale ranges from 1 to 14. The chemistry of acids and bases doesn't necessarily fit what we imagine this scale to be and so it is possible to have acids that dip into negative figures, although we would not want to find these in the human body.

pH relates to the amount of hydrogen ions in aqueous solution. It is always a small p before the H because small ps denote either potential or partial pressure as a convention. Hydrogen is an atom that has one proton (which is positive) and one electron (which is negative) and one neutron (which is neutrally charged and which we will now ignore for the rest of this explanation).

pH stands for 'potential of hydrogen'. This is the potential of something to release hydrogen ions. From our previous explanation we can see that hydrogen can only become an **ion** when it transfers an electron, which is negative. That leaves hydrogen with one proton, in fact all it is now is a proton (and the neutron which we aren't concerned with) which is positive. So, hydrogen ions are denoted H⁺ and the greater number of them you have the more acidic something will be. This then explains the name of the drugs which reduce stomach acid called **proton pump inhibitors**, abbreviated as PPIs. PPIs stop the production and pumping of protons by parietal cells into the stomach.

Pure water is pH neutral, 7, whilst acids have a pH range of 0–6.9 and bases (alkalis) 7.1–14 (see Figure 1.3). Figure 1.4 illustrates everyday items on the pH scale.

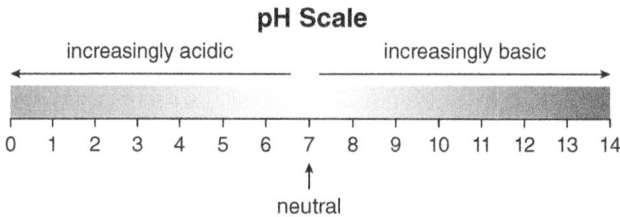

**Figure 1.3**  pH scale

## Principles of Water and Body Fluid Compartments

The human body is made up mostly of water. This is important as the chemical reactions of life take place within aqueous solutions. The percentage of water varies depending upon age and sex, ranging from approximately 75% of body mass in infants to 60% in adult males and 55% in adult females, which can further decrease to as low as 45% in old age.

Luckily, water is compartmentalised within our tissues to prevent us from looking like a big water balloon! Each compartment is largely separated from another by a physical barrier. In the human body, water is distributed into two main compartments:

*Intracellular fluid (ICF)*, which is the totality of fluid enclosed in cells by their plasma membrane, compromising approximately 60% of the body's total water content

*Extracellular fluid (ECF)*, which is the totality of fluid found outside the cell

In total, a 70 kg male has 45 litres of body water, but it is important to understand in which compartment this water is held (see Figure 1.5).

INTRODUCING PHARMACOLOGY | 11

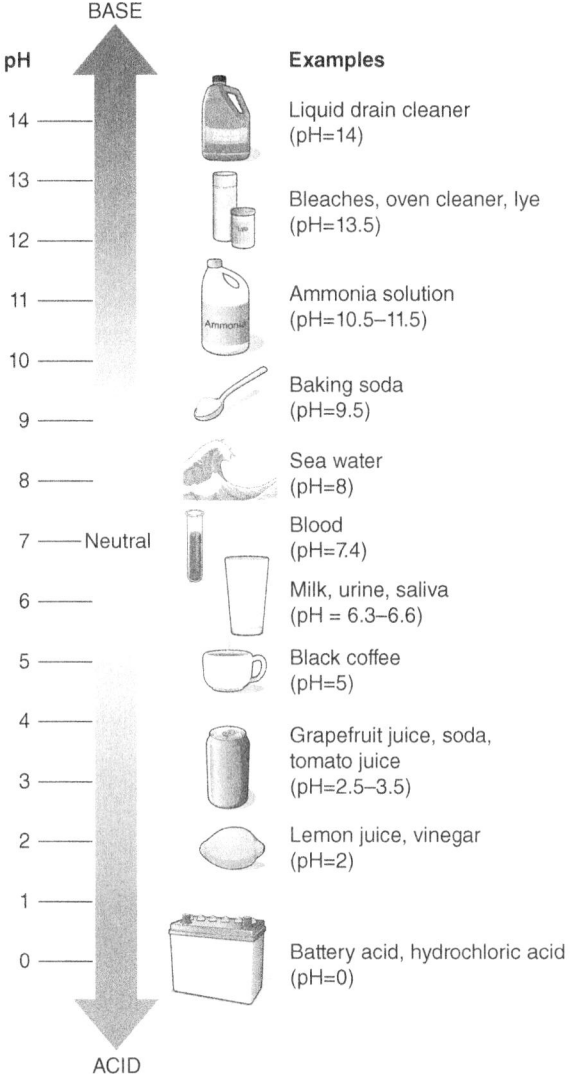

**Figure 1.4** Everyday items on the pH scale

*Source*: Rice University. Licensed under a Creative Commons Attribution 4.0 International License.

| Adult male: Total body water volume = 45 litres (approximately 60% of body weight) ||| 
|---|---|---|
| Intracellular fluid volume = 30 litres | Extracellular fluid volume = 15 litres (approximately 20% of body weight) ||
| | Interstitial fluid volume = 10 litres | Plasma volume = 5 litres |

**Figure 1.5** Total body water volume for an adult male

ECF surrounds all cells in the body and accounts for one third of the body's water content. It has two primary components: the fluid part of the blood called *plasma* and the *interstitial fluid* (IF) that surrounds all cells that are not in the blood. Plasma transports a range of materials such as blood cells, proteins, electrolytes, nutrients, gases and waste materials via the blood vessels. Nutrients, gases and waste materials travel between capillaries and cells through the IF. Cells are separated from the extracellular fluid compartment by a selectively permeable cell membrane that helps regulate the passage of materials between this space and the inside of the cell.

The body also has other water-based ECF compartments such as cerebrospinal fluid which surrounds the brain and spinal cord, lymph, synovial fluid in joints, pleural fluid in the pleural cavities, pericardial fluid in the cardiac sac, peritoneal fluid in the peritoneal cavity, and the aqueous humour of the eye (see Figure 1.6).

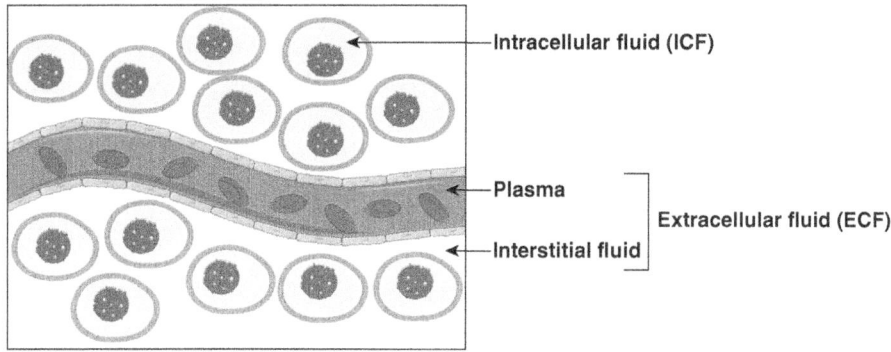

**Figure 1.6** Water distribution

*Source*: Created using Servier Medical Art. Servial Medical Art is licenced under CC BY 4.0: https://creativecommons.org/licenses/by/4.0

Although we are talking about water here, it is not pure water, but a mixture of dissolved substances known as **solutes**, which are deemed important to sustain life. These solutes include electrolytes. Electrolytes are substances that separate into charged ions when they are dissolved in water. For example, sodium chloride (table salt) separates into sodium (Na$^+$) and chloride (Cl$^-$) ions in water.

Electrolytes, important in basic physiological functioning, originate from food. Elevated or low levels of electrolytes can affect normal bodily functions and may lead to life-threatening conditions. Therefore, it is essential to maintain the homeostatic balance of electrolytes and water inside and outside the cells. The cell membrane is selectively permeable, which means the movement of electrolytes and other substances across the membrane can be regulated. Whilst electrolytes require specific channels, transport proteins and sometimes energy to cross cell membranes, water moves freely by the process of **osmosis**.

Some of the most significant electrolytes are sodium, potassium, chloride, magnesium, calcium, phosphate and bicarbonates, and we will now explore these functions in a little more depth.

The concentration of these electrolytes is different in the ICF and ECF (see Table 1.3).

**Table 1.4** Concentration of electrolytes

| Ion | Intracellular concentration (mMol) | Extracellular concentration (mMol) |
| --- | --- | --- |
| Sodium Na$^+$ | 15 | 142 |
| Potassium K$^+$ | 150 | 4.0 |
| Calcium Ca$^{2+}$ | 10$^{-4}$ | 1 |

## Sodium

Sodium is one of the essential electrolytes in the extracellular fluid. Sodium ions are involved in maintaining the extracellular fluid volume. For example, a person who exercises excessively will lose both water and sodium through sweat. In response, they may drink large amounts of water which enters the bloodstream and risks diluting the remaining sodium in the blood. The concentration of sodium falls, a condition known as hyponatraemia. If this imbalance is prolonged, water moves through osmosis from the blood into cells, the cells swell and rupture.

Conversely, if the same person is exercising excessively and not replacing lost water and electrolytes by drinking fluids, this may lead to increased sodium levels in the blood or hypernatraemia. This high concentration of sodium in the extracellular fluid will cause water to leave cells by osmosis, making them shrink.

Deranged sodium levels, independent of the cause, will trigger homeostatic processes. In hypernatraemia for example, osmoreceptors in the hypothalamus detect the increased concentration of the blood and activate homeostatic responses which include thirst and reduction of urine output.

## Potassium

Potassium ions are found in increased concentrations in the intracellular fluid. Along with sodium ions, they are involved in regulating the membrane potential of cells, which is particularly important in nerve conduction.

A membrane potential is the voltage across the cell membrane. Cells do not like sodium because of the potential to disrupt fluid movement across the cell membrane. Sodium–potassium pumps (see **active transport**) are located in the cell membrane and use energy, in the form of adenosine triphosphate (ATP), to actively move sodium ions out of the cell, whilst pumping potassium in. For each pair of potassium ions that are moved into the cell, three sodium ions are moved out, and this causes an overall loss of positive charge from the cell resulting in a negative charge inside the cell relative to the outside. This is constant when the cell is at rest (see Figure 1.7).

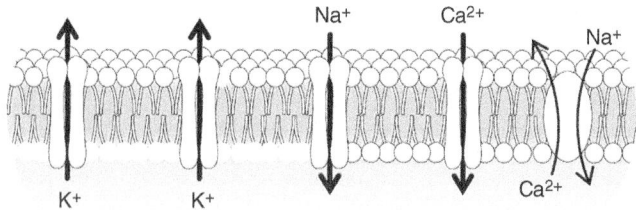

**Figure 1.7** Cell membrane

### Chloride

Chloride ions are negatively charged ions (anions) found mainly in the extracellular fluid. They are a significant contributor to the osmotic pressure gradient between the ICF and ECF. Chloride is involved in regulation of water movement between ICF and ECF to maintain proper hydration.

### Calcium

Calcium ions are extracellular positive ions (cations) and enter cells by specific calcium channels and transporters. They are the major signalling ions in cells, playing a vital role in many physiological functions of the body including skeletal mineralisation, contraction of muscles, regulation of heartbeat, blood clotting and secretion of hormones. Just like sodium and potassium, calcium also has a significant role in neurotransmission.

### Phosphate

Phosphate is present in the body in three ionic forms, calcium phosphate $Ca_3(PO_4)_2$, dihydrogen phosphate ($H_2PO_4$) and mono hydrogen phosphate ($HPO_4$). Phosphate is found in **phospholipids**, such as those that make up the cell membrane, and in ATP, nucleotides and buffers. Buffers are substances that have a neutralising effect on hydrogen ions. They help maintain the body at the correct pH so that biochemical processes continue to run optimally.

Most of the phosphate (along with calcium) that enters the body is incorporated into bones and teeth, and bone serves as a mineral reserve for these ions.

### Bicarbonate

Bicarbonate is the second most abundant anion in the blood. Alongside phosphate ions, bicarbonate ions are also part of the body's buffer systems to help maintain the body's acid–base balance.

Up to three-quarters of the carbon dioxide in the human body is converted to carbonic acid, which is quickly converted to bicarbonate in the cytoplasm of red blood cells. Bicarbonate is transported in the blood. Once it reaches the lungs, the reaction is reversed and carbon dioxide is regenerated from bicarbonate to be exhaled as metabolic waste.

If bicarbonate levels are too high or too low, then this can suggest that the body is struggling to maintain its acid–base buffering system. This could be caused by an electrolyte imbalance or the inability to remove the waste product carbon dioxide from the body.

### Enzymes

Enzymes are proteins that speed up biochemical reactions, frequently defined as biological catalysts. Catalysts are substances that increase the rate of a chemical reaction but do not undergo any change themselves. This is useful as it means they can be used repeatedly. Almost all metabolic processes within the cell require enzyme action. Some examples of these metabolic processes involve the digestion of food to prepare for absorption whilst others are involved in detoxification processes in the liver. The role of the liver in drug metabolism will be explored in Chapter 4.

Enzymes will usually only catalyse one specific reaction (although some may catalyse several types), so this means there is a huge array of enzymes within the body. The molecule entering the reaction is called the **substrate**, and this binds to the active site of the enzyme. Whilst the substrate is bound to the active site, the reaction occurs. Once this is complete the product (or products) of the reaction is released from the active site and the enzyme will be used again. Enzymes can catalyse the combination of two or more substrates into a larger product (anabolic reaction) or break down substrates into smaller products (catabolic reactions).

Figure 1.8 illustrates the products of enzyme-catalysed reaction. Note that the enzyme remains unchanged as products of the enzyme-catalysed reaction leave the active site of the enzyme.

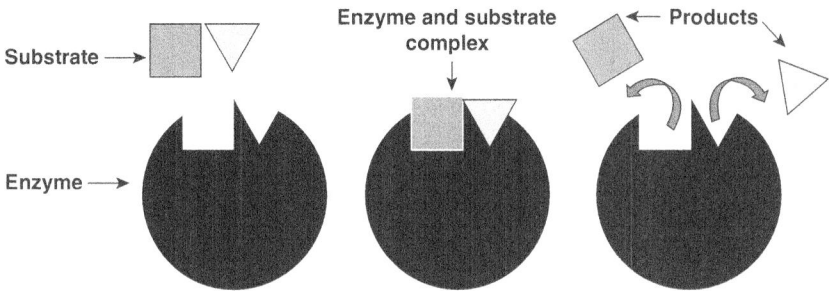

**Figure 1.8** Products of enzyme-catalysed reaction

Most enzymes are named by adding the suffix -ase after the substrate they act upon.

**Lipases:** This is a group of enzymes, produced in the pancreas, stomach and salivary glands, involved in fat digestion.

*Amylase*: An enzyme secreted by the salivary glands and pancreas which converts dietary starches into sugars

*Maltase*: Also present in the saliva and converts sugar maltose into glucose

*Trypsin*: These enzymes are present in the small intestine and convert dietary proteins into amino acids

*Lactase*: These enzymes break down lactose, the sugar in milk, into glucose and galactose

*Acetylcholinesterase*: These enzymes break down the neurotransmitter acetylcholine at the neuromuscular junction

Enzymes will only work under certain conditions. Most enzymes act optimally at 37 degrees Celsius, the body's temperature. If the enzymes are exposed to lower temperatures, they may work more slowly. Different enzymes tolerate various levels of acidity. For example, enzymes in the intestines work best at a pH of 8 and those in the stomach at a pH between 1 and 2. This is because the stomach is more acidic. If enzymes are exposed to extremes of pH or high temperatures, the shape of their active site may change. If this happens then the substrate will no longer fit into the enzymes, and we say that the enzyme has been denatured.

A cofactor, an additional chemical component, is sometimes bound to enzymes and required for enzymatic activity. A cofactor may be either an ion or small molecule (e.g. a vitamin) but some enzymes require both.

It is important to understand the activity of enzymes in catalysing biochemical reactions as many drugs are developed which either inhibit or induce enzyme action. These concepts are explained in Chapter 6.

## Cell Structure and Function

The human body contains trillions of cells, and they provide structure and support. Cells are the smallest units of the body and are responsible for all its physiological functions and processes.

Cells come in a variety of shapes and sizes depending on their function. However, there are three main parts to all cells: the cell membrane, the cytoplasm and the nucleus (except the erythrocyte, red blood cell, which does not contain nuclei).

It is important to understand the structure and function of cells as many drugs manipulate cell activity.

Figure 1.9 illustrates the important parts of the cell, and we will briefly explore the functions of each part.

### Nucleus

A nucleus is the cell's headquarters. It is the largest and most visible of all cell structures and contains the body's genetic material. The nucleus is contained within a nuclear envelope which contains pores to allow substances to pass between it and the cytoplasm. Within the nucleus is the nucleolus, a spherical structure that is involved in the production and assembly of ribosomes.

INTRODUCING PHARMACOLOGY | 17

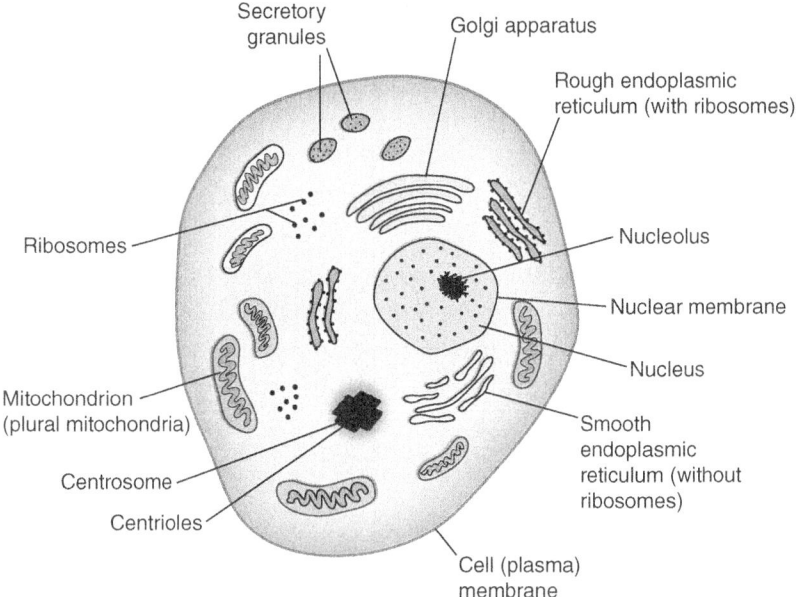

**Figure 1.9** Important parts of the cell

## Cytoplasm

The cytoplasm is the inside of the cell that surrounds the nucleus. It makes up most of the cell's volume and contains the organelles within a jelly-like fluid – cytosol. Many important cellular reactions take place in the cytoplasm.

## Mitochondria

Mitochondria are membranous, sausage-like structures and are often known as the powerhouses of the cell. They help turn energy from food into energy in the form of ATP.

## Ribosomes

Ribosomes are tiny granules that are made of both ribonucleic acid (RNA) and protein. They are found on the outer surface of the rough endoplasmic reticulum and are also scattered throughout the cytoplasm. Ribosomes synthesise proteins from amino acids using RNA as a template and are known as the 'protein factories'. These proteins include the enzymes required for metabolism.

## Endoplasmic Reticulum

Endoplasmic reticulum (ER) is a series of interconnecting membranous canals in the cytoplasm and is connected to the nuclear envelope that surrounds the nucleus. It can be either rough or smooth. Smooth ER synthesises lipids and steroid hormones and its enzymes are involved in detoxification of some drugs. Rough ER is studded with ribosomes. Proteins are made here and then transported to the Golgi complex for further processing. The rough ER is the cell's membrane factory as it makes vital proteins and phospholipids that form part of the cell membrane.

## Golgi Complex/Golgi Apparatus

The Golgi apparatus consists of stacks of closely folded and flattened membranous sacs. The Golgi apparatus is often thought of as the post office of the cell as it processes and packages proteins and lipid molecules. These are later transported to other cell compartments or secreted from the cell.

## Lysosomes

Lysosomes are small organelles that dispose of cell waste. They are specialised vesicles that provide a protected environment for potentially dangerous chemical reactions. They use powerful enzymes to break down foreign materials that may have entered the cell. They ingest and dissolve unwanted cell parts and either dispose of or recycle them.

## Centrioles

Centrioles help chromosomes move inside the cell. During cell division, the centrioles form a spindle-shaped structure essential for movement of the DNA strands.

## Microtubules

Microtubules are hollow tubes constructed from a protein called tubulin. They provide structure for the cell by anchoring the organelles. They also help change the shape of the cell when they disassemble. Microtubules also aid movement of vesicles and organelles within the cell. They are usually found on absorptive cell surfaces such as the intestines.

## Microvilli

Microvilli are microscopic finger-like protrusions on the cellular membrane that help increase surface area for **diffusion**. They are usually found on absorptive cell surfaces such as the intestines.

## Vacuole (or Vesicles)

A vacuole is a chamber surrounded by a **semi-permeable** membrane which only lets certain molecules through. It keeps the cytosol from being exposed to the contents inside. Vacuoles are used whenever a large amount of substance is taken into the cell by **endocytosis**, or out of the cell by **exocytosis**. Endocytosis and exocytosis are explained further in the section on bulk transport later in this chapter.

## Plasma Membrane

The plasma membrane (see Figure 1.10) defines the boundaries of the cell. It separates and protects the interior of the cell from the external environment. It is made up of a bilayer of phospholipids (see Figure 1.11). The phospholipids have an electrically charged head which is **hydrophilic** (water loving) and a tail which has no charge and is hydrophobic (water hating).

INTRODUCING PHARMACOLOGY | 19

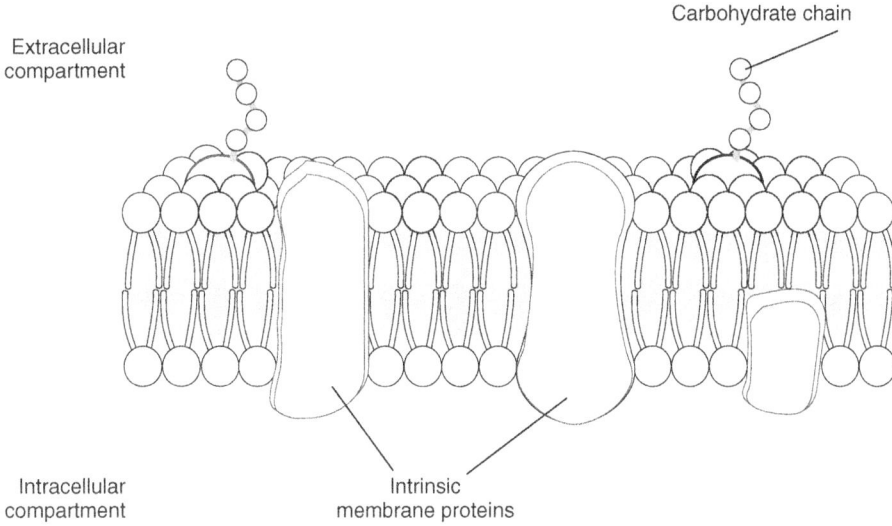

**Figure 1.10** Plasma membrane

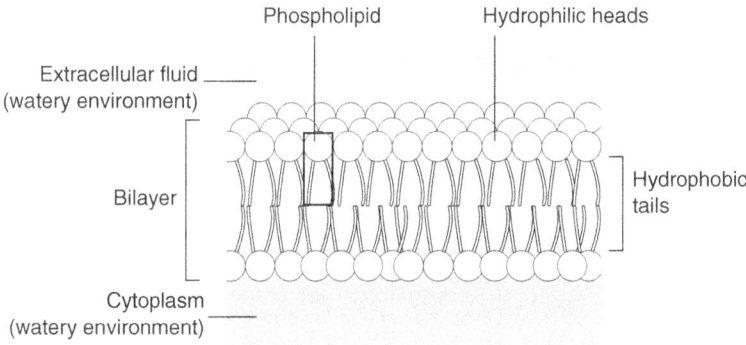

**Figure 1.11** Phospholipids

The plasma membrane also contains proteins, some of which span the width of the membrane acting as channels and some are located on the surface. These proteins have a variety of functions:

- Enzyme activity
- Self-markers, providing the cell with immunological identity
- Receptors for chemical messengers including hormones
- Formation of channels to allow substances to cross the membrane
- Involved with pumps to help transport substances across the membrane

The plasma membrane is selectively permeable to allow some substances through but not others and regulate the cell's internal environment. The cell membrane does this through either active or passive mechanisms. Active and passive transport mechanisms will now be further explored.

## Transport of Substances Across Cell Membranes

There are three passive mechanisms through which substances move across cell membranes.

### Diffusion

Diffusion is the movement of molecules from an area of high concentration to an area of low concentration (the concentration gradient) and this can occur across a semi-permeable membrane. This process does not require any energy. Once particles have diffused, they are evenly distributed and reach a state of equilibrium as illustrated in Figure 1.12.

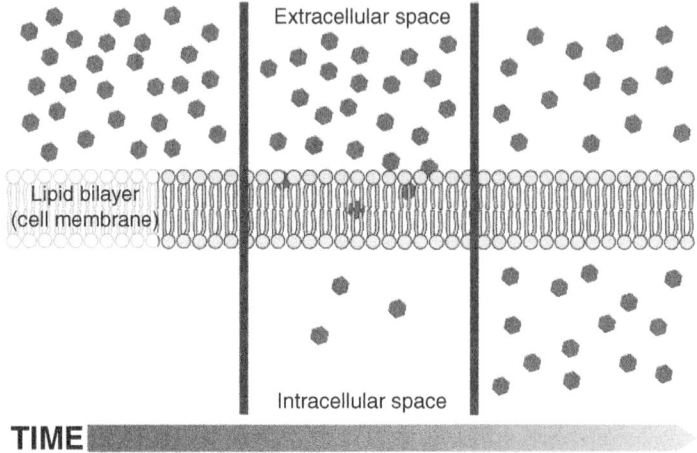

**Figure 1.12** Different ways molecules move in cells

*Source*: Wikimedia Commons under the Creative Commons CC0 License

Substances will only diffuse across the cell membrane if the membrane is permeable to the substance and if the concentration is higher on one side of the membrane than the other. The properties of the substances are significant. Small or lipid soluble particles can easily diffuse through the plasma membrane (e.g. oxygen and fat-soluble vitamins). Oxygen continuously diffuses from blood into cells as the concentration is always higher in the blood than the tissues. Fat soluble vitamins readily pass through the plasma membrane in the digestive tract.

Some substances (e.g. glucose, amino acids), however, require help by carrier proteins to pass through the cell's lipid bilayer, known as facilitated diffusion. Substances either bind to a carrier protein in the cell membrane and then move across it or move through water-filled protein channels.

### Osmosis

This is a special type of diffusion where water molecules diffuse from an area of higher water concentration to an area of lower water concentration. This is usually because other molecules present are too large to diffuse across the membrane. Solutions which contain higher concentrations of solutes have a lower concentration of water molecules and vice versa. Therefore, water will diffuse towards an area with higher solute concentrations. The ability of osmosis to create enough force to 'pull' the water from a dilute solution to a more concentrated solution is called 'osmotic pressure'. Via osmosis, water equilibrates throughout the body and concentration of water and solutes is almost the same in intracellular and extracellular fluid. The concentration may be the same, but the volume may be different (see Figure 1.13).

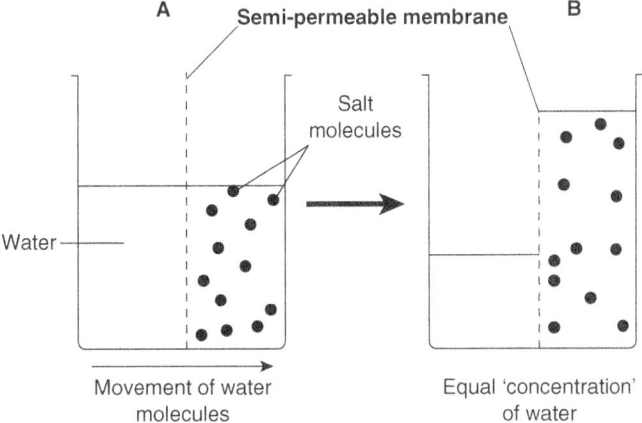

**Figure 1.13** How water equilibrates via osmosis

The solute concentration in body compartments will influence the direction of water movement through osmosis (see Figure 1.14). An isotonic solution, *iso* meaning 'the same', has the same concentration as the inside of a cell, so there is no overall net movement of water. If, however, a cell is placed in a hypotonic solution (i.e. a solution which holds more water (less solute) than inside the cell), the net movement of water will be to the inside of the cell. This will increase the water content inside the cell and risks cell rupture. Alternatively, if a cell is suspended in a hypertonic solution, it holds less water (more solute) and water will move from the inside of the cell to the extracellular compartment. The cell will shrink and become crenated.

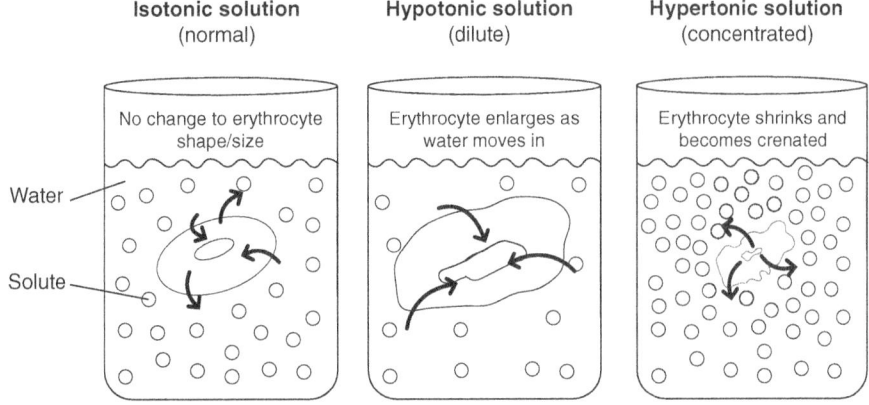

**Figure 1.14** Solute concentration in body compartments

## Filtration

This is the movement of water and solutes through a membrane due to hydrostatic pressure from the cardiovascular system. For example, blood being filtered in the glomerulus of the kidney to retain essential substances which can then be reabsorbed.

While passive mechanisms such as filtration rely on concentration gradients, the body also employs active and bulk transport processes to move substances across membranes, often requiring energy expenditure to achieve these essential functions.

## Active Transport

Active transport is the movement of particles through membranes from regions of lower concentrations to higher concentrations (see Figure 1.15). Like facilitated diffusion, it also requires carrier proteins but unlike facilitated diffusion, active transport requires energy in the form of ATP (see Figure 1.16). One of the most studied active transport systems is the sodium–potassium pump. As discussed earlier, potassium levels are much higher inside the cell and sodium levels are much higher outside the cell. These ions tend to diffuse down their concentration gradients, potassium outwards and sodium inwards. To maintain their concentration gradients, excess sodium is constantly pumped out of the cell in exchange for potassium.

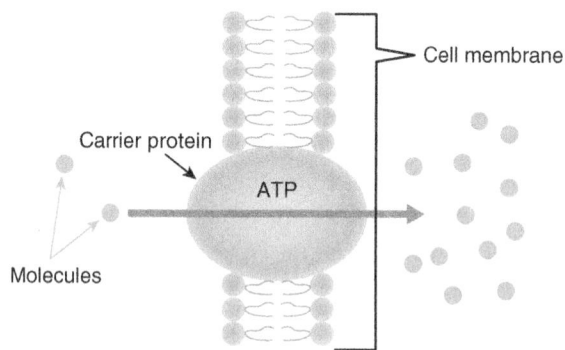

**Figure 1.15** Active transport

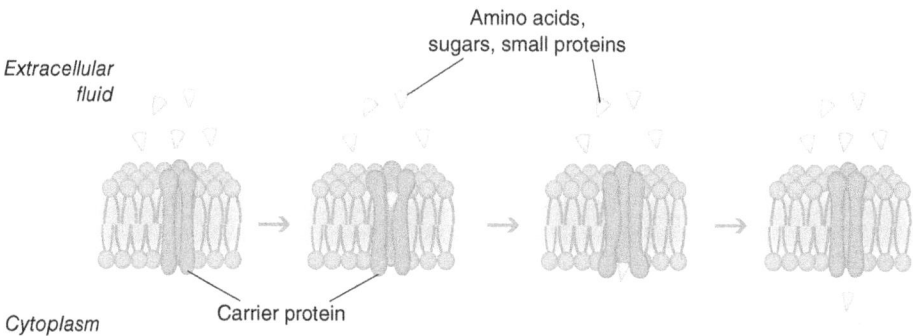

**Figure 1.16** Carrier proteins

## Bulk Transport

This involves the transportation of large particles and macromolecules that are too big to cross the cell membrane via vesicles. They also require energy from ATP. Bulk transport is divided into two types: endocytosis and exocytosis (see Figure 1.17).

Endocytosis involves pinocytosis or 'cell drinking' and phagocytosis 'cell-eating'. Pinocytosis allows the cell to bring in fluid by engulfing it with the extension of the cytoplasm of the cell, whilst phagocytosis involves taking in solids instead of liquids. Lysosomes then attach to the vesicles and release enzymes to digest the contents.

Exocytosis is the opposite process to endocytosis, where the substance stored in a vesicle is secreted from the cell. The vesicle migrates towards the membrane and attaches itself to it. It then ruptures and its contents are emptied outside the cell. Exocytosis is involved in hormone and mucous secretion and neurotransmitter release.

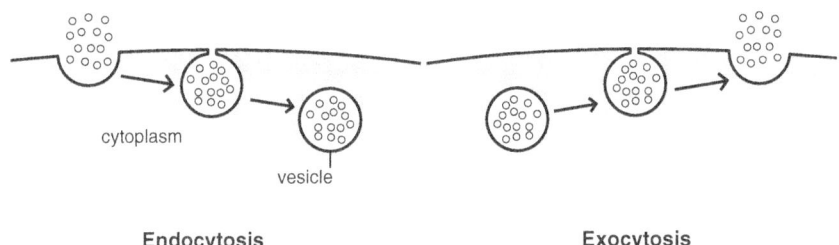

**Figure 1.17** Bulk transport

---

### PAUSE AND REFLECT 1.3

Review the different mechanisms of cell transport and for each, provide an example.

---

## Cell Function

Cells are highly specialised in terms of both structure and function.
The main functions of cells are:

*Movement*: This is provided by muscle cells which can generate forces to produce movement.

*Conductivity*: This is the primary function of the nerve cell. Conduction is a response to a stimulus which causes a wave of excitation, enabling an electrical potential to move across the cell's surface to reach other parts.

*Metabolic absorption*: All cells take in and use other substances from their surroundings. Cells of the kidney's tubules reabsorb fluids and synthesise proteins. This will be looked at in more detail in Chapter 5.

*Secretion*: Certain cells can create (synthesise) new substances from those they absorb. These new substances are secreted to be used wherever they are needed. For example, cells of the adrenal glands (located on the kidneys), ovaries and testes secrete hormonal steroids.

*Excretion*: All cells excrete waste products, which is the process of removing undesirable end products following the metabolism of nutrients.

*Respiration*: All cells take in oxygen as they require this to change nutrients into energy in the form of adenosine triphosphate (ATP). This takes place in the mitochondria.

*Reproduction*: Cells form tissue as they enlarge and reproduce themselves. Tissue requires maintenance by new cells replacing those cells that are ageing and programmed to self-destruct. Cells reproduce by a process called mitosis, which involves the cell dividing and forming two genetically identical daughter cells. The only exception to this is the gamete or sex cells which are formed through a process called meiosis.

*Communication*: This is essential for cells to survive, connect and create a solid, well-formed organism. Constant communication leads to the maintenance of a dynamic, steady state. Any breakdown in communication can lead to disease and so it is tightly regulated. We will now explore cell communication a little further.

## Sending and Receiving of Signals

As previously stated, the cells of our bodies are also constantly receiving signals from other cells which are important to keep cells alive and functioning. For example, cells may need to send messages to their neighbours such as 'I need oxygen' or 'Please help, I am being invaded by a virus.' The process involves the first cell (A) sending a signal molecule to the receiving cell (B). These signal molecules are called ligands and are often chemicals that can be found in the extracellular fluid surrounding cells such as proteins, lipids, hormones, growth factors or even neurotransmitters. Cell B needs a receptor so that the signalling molecule can bind to it.

The signals can be grouped into different categories defined by the distance they travel to reach the receiving cell (see Figure 1.18).

## Autocrine

Cells may produce signals which bind to receptors on their own surface, making it possible to send messages to themselves. This is called autocrine signalling, and while it sounds a little strange that a cell would want to communicate with itself, it is essential during development as it ensures correct cell division and maintaining cell identity.

## Juxtacrine

Cells in direct contact or those that are situated close to each other can be connected by gap junctions which are protein channels. This enables signalling molecules to easily pass through these junctions to neighbouring cells, allowing groups of cells to respond to a signal received by just one cell.

### Paracrine

Paracrine signalling happens between two nearby cells that are not connected. The signalling molecules in this case diffuse across short distances to pass the message on. Communication between neurons is a notable example of this. Neurons release neurotransmitters into a gap known as a synapse so that the message can be passed onto the next.

### Endocrine

These signalling molecules need to travel through the tissues and bloodstream to reach their target destination. The signals are hormones – for example, thyroid-stimulating hormone, which is produced and released into the bloodstream by the pituitary gland and targets the thyroid gland that releases thyroid hormones essential for stimulating the metabolic rate of the body.

Once the cell receives the incoming signals, the cell responds by activating a variety of transduction pathways.

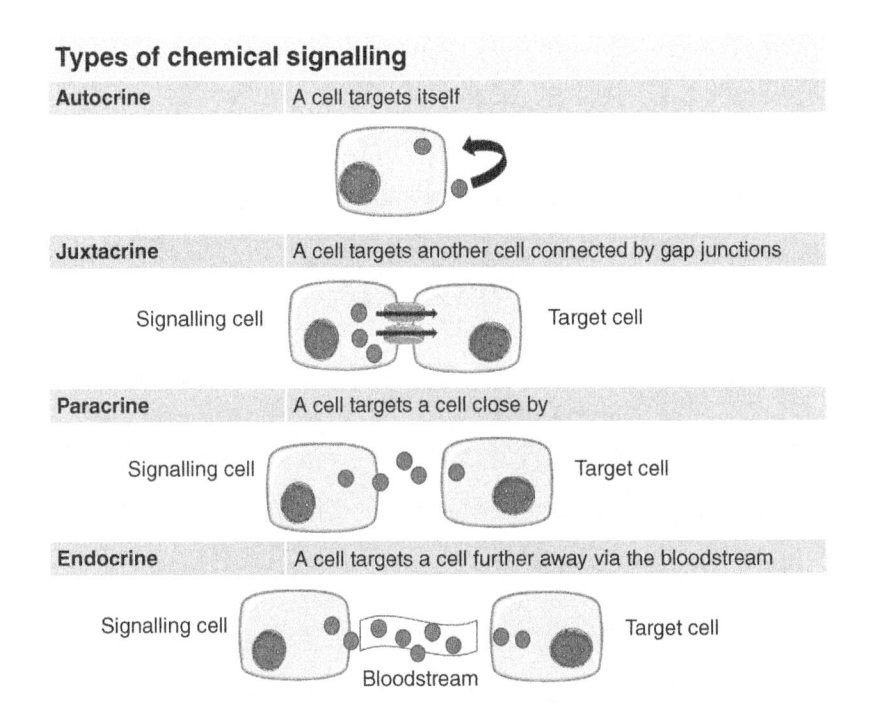

**Figure 1.18** Types of chemical signalling

Source: Created using Servier Medical Art. Servier Medical Art is licenced under https://creativecommons.org/licenses/by/3.0/

## Transduction

These pathways often involve the addition or removal of phosphate groups, which results in the activation of proteins. Enzymes that transfer phosphate groups from ATP to a protein are called protein kinases. Many of the relay molecules in a signal transduction pathway are protein kinases and often act on other protein kinases in the pathway. Often this creates a phosphorylation cascade, where one enzyme phosphorylates another, which then phosphorylates another protein, causing a chain reaction. These chain reactions have essential functions:

- They physically transfer the signal from where it was received to another part of the cell where the response is expected.
- They amplify the signal received, making it much stronger.
- They distribute the signal so that it influences several processes concurrently being relayed to several different targets within the cell, causing a complex response.
- The signal can be changed by another factor that occurs inside or outside the cell.

It is also important to acknowledge the role of protein phosphatases on the phosphorylation cascade. These are a group of enzymes that can quickly remove phosphate groups from proteins (dephosphorylation) and so inactivate protein kinases. This action 'turns off' the signal transduction pathway, which is vital to ensure that the cellular response is regulated appropriately. Dephosphorylation also makes protein kinases available for reuse and enables the cell to respond again when another signal is received.

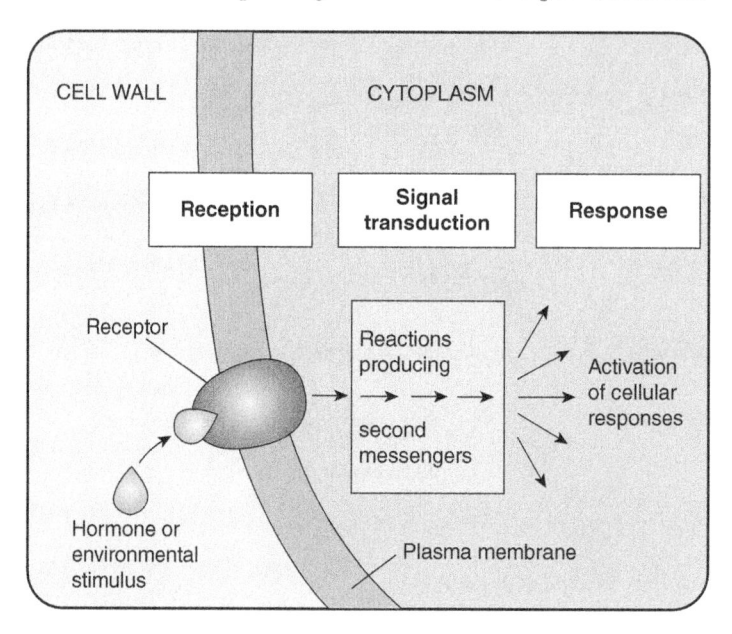

**Figure 1.19** Signal transduction pathways model

*Source*: Wikipedia under the Creative Commons license.

Kinases are not the only tools used by cells in signal transduction. Small, nonprotein, water-soluble molecules or ions called second messengers (the **ligand** that binds to the receptor being the first messenger) can also relay signals received by receptors on the cell surface to target molecules in the cytoplasm or the nucleus. Examples of second messengers include cyclic adenosine monophosphate (cAMP) and calcium ions.

Once a signal reaches its target molecule, it can change the cell's behaviour. The cell can respond by growing, dividing, differentiating or even dying via a process called apoptosis (see Figure 1.19).

## Cell Cycle

The lifespan or life cycle of a cell describes the time it remains functional before it undergoes programmed cell death or is replaced through cell division. The lifespan of a cell is cyclical rather than a linear pathway, because the original cell (or mother cell) grows and then divides to make two cells (daughter cells). These daughter cells then start exactly the same process over again from the beginning.

The life cycle of a cell undergoes certain sequential stages which are divided into two major phases: interphase and the mitotic (M) phase.

The interphase comprises three phases: G1, S and G2.

1.  *G1 (growth 1 or gap phase 1)*: During this phase, the cell grows and increases in size. It does not replicate DNA in this phase but carries out its normal cellular functions. Some cells exit the cycle after G1 phase and do not divide again, such as muscle cells and neurons. This is called G0 phase, where they remain metabolically active but do not divide again unless called upon to do so – for example, to replace any damaged cells or those lost to cell death.
2.  *S phase (synthesis phase)*: Once the cell has grown to a stage where it is no longer functioning well, it needs to divide. In the S phase, the cell's DNA is replicated.
3.  *G2 (growth 2 or gap phase 2)*: The cell undergoes further changes ready for division.

*The mitotic (M) phase* consists of mitosis which is the division of the nucleus followed by cytokinesis, the division of the cytoplasm. Mitosis consists of five basic phases: prophase, prometaphase, metaphase, anaphase and telophase. Cytokinesis starts in anaphase or telophase. See Figure 1.20 for further explanation of what happens within the cell during these phases. At the end of the mitotic phase there are two daughter cells that are identical to each other and the original mother cell.

Throughout the cell lifespan, cells use special proteins and 'checkpoint' signalling systems to regulate the progression of the cell life cycle. Checkpoints exist at the end of G1 and at the beginning of G2 phases and to check for damage to DNA before and after S phase. There is a further checkpoint during mitosis too. If there is any damage to the DNA the cell is forced to undergo cell death or apoptosis. This is important as cancers may occur when cells with damaged DNA reproduce. Thus, checking to see if a cell's DNA has been damaged immediately before replication helps reduce the risk of cancers developing. Drugs used to treat cancer will be explored in Chapter 6.

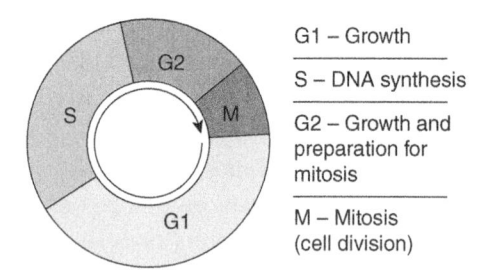

**Figure 1.20** The four phases of the cell cycle: G1 - the initial growth phase. S - the phase in which DNA is synthesised. G2 - the second growth phase in preparation for cell division. M - mitosis; where the cell divides to produce two daughter cells that continue the cell cycle.

*Source*: Created using Servier Medical Art. Servier Medical Art is licenced under Creative Commons Attribution-Share Alike 3.0

## CHAPTER SUMMARY

Chapter 1 has explored several biochemical, anatomical and physiological principles which are necessary to sustain cellular, tissue and organ function. The body maintains these processes through specialised cellular signalling, processes and communication. When these functions are compromised and disease results, drugs may be required to restore homeostasis. Drugs will also need to move across cell membranes to have an effect and they do this by a variety of mechanisms such as diffusion, osmosis, **filtration** and active transportation. The control of ions between extracellular and intracellular fluid compartments is also important in maintaining the body's physiological functions, and drugs are developed to alter the movement of the ions mentioned.

The function of enzymes is also explored. Enzymes act to increase the rate of chemical reactions and some drugs act to inhibit enzyme activity. Enzymes will only work in certain environments, including temperature and pH. pH is the measure of an acidity or basicity of a solution and refers to the concentraion of hydrogen ions in a solution. pH can affect the physiological processes in our body and is also significant for the action of drugs and how they are absorbed, distributed and excreted.

# ROUTES OF DRUG ADMINISTRATION AND DRUG ABSORPTION

# 2

---
### LEARNING OUTCOMES
---

By the end of this chapter, you should be able to:

1. Describe the anatomical structures and physiological processes relevant to the routes of drug administration
2. Explore the different routes of drug administration
3. Critically appraise the factors which affect the rate and extent of drug absorption

## INTRODUCTION

Chapter 2 will explore the various routes of drug administration, the normal physiology relevant to the mode of drug administration and examine the advantages, disadvantages and considerations for each route as applied to safe and therapeutic medicine management.

The first stage of the pharmacokinetic process is *drug absorption*, defined as the movement of the drug from the site of administration into the systemic circulation. This is important so that the drug is transferred to its intended site of action and can exert its clinical effect.

It is important to note, however, that there are several groups of drugs which do not require absorption because their mode of action occurs within the cavity they have been directly administered into. Examples include the instillation of medication to the eye to treat infection and **laxatives** or anti-diarrhoea medications.

The factors which affect the rate and extent of drug absorption can be categorised in two ways. Firstly, factors which relate to the *physio-chemical properties of the drug* and secondly the different *anatomical and physiological characteristics of the human body*.

The routes of drug administration are summarised as:

1. **Enteral**
   i. Oral
   ii. Rectal
2. **Buccal**
3. **Sublingual**
4. **Topical**
5. **Transdermal**
6. **Parenteral**
   i. **Subcutaneous**
   ii. **Intramuscular**
   iii. **Intravenous**
   iv. Intra-arterial
   v. Intraosseous
7. Inhalation

# THE ENTERAL ROUTE OF DRUG ADMINISTRATION

The enteral route refers to the administration of drug into the gastrointestinal system.

The most common enteral route of drug administration is the oral route with over 80% of medications administered in this way, primarily because it is convenient, with oral dosage forms deemed relatively simple and cost effective to manufacture compared to other routes of administration.

The gastrointestinal tract anatomically comprises many sections, and therefore multiple physiological factors influence the rate and extent of the absorption of drugs.

The gastrointestinal tract is a muscular tube, measuring approximately 9 metres from the mouth to the anus in the adult, and has varying diameters along its length. The gastrointestinal tract is a complicated system, with each organ containing multiple distinct tissues dedicated to digesting food efficiently while preventing non-food molecules from entering pre-systemic circulation (see Figure 2.1).

It extends from the mouth to the anus and is divided into four distinct anatomical regions:

1. The oesophageal sphincter
2. The stomach (cardia, fundus, corpus, antrum, pylorus)
3. The small intestine (duodenum, jejunum, ileum)
4. The large intestine (colorectum)

The tube's inner luminal surface is extremely uneven, which increases the surface area available for absorption. The wall of the gastrointestinal tract is essentially identical along its length, consisting of four major layers (see Figure 2.2).

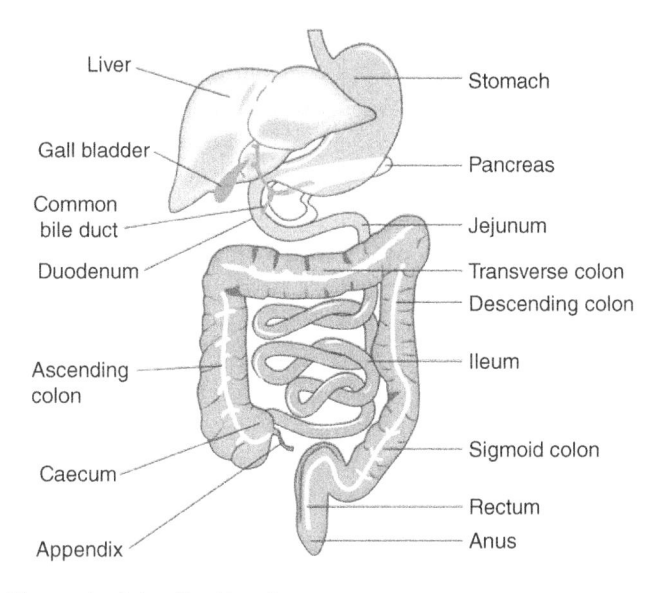

# ROUTES OF DRUG ADMINISTRATION AND DRUG ABSORPTION | 31

**Figure 2.1** The gastrointestinal tract

1. The serosa – the outer layer of epithelium
2. The muscularis externa comprised of three layers of smooth muscle, two inner layers with circular fibres and a thin outer layer that runs longitudinally. These muscles contract to provide contractions to move the gastrointestinal contents and physically break it down
3. The submucosa – a connective tissue layer rich in blood and lymphatic vessels that contains some secretory tissue and nerves
4. The mucosa

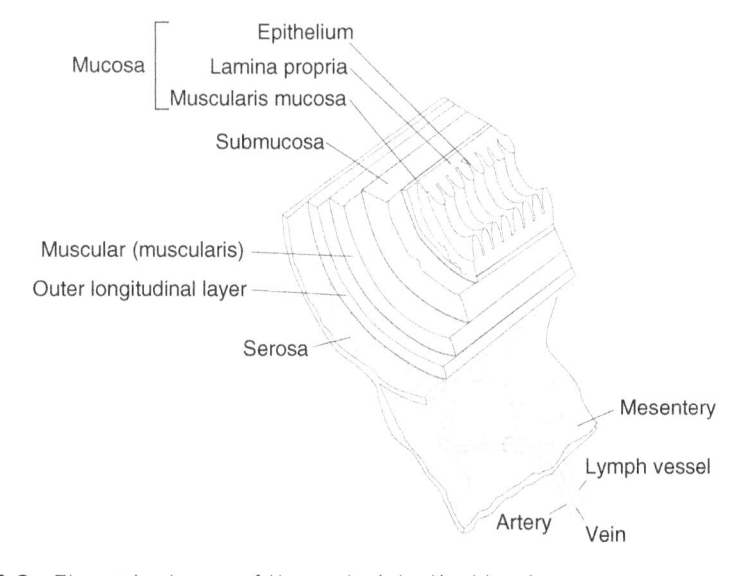

**Figure 2.2** The major layers of the gastrointestinal tract

Most of the gastrointestinal epithelium is mucous coated (mucous: adjective and mucus: noun). This is a sticky, clear mucin-water complex that is secreted as a protective layer and mechanical barrier in the gastrointestinal tract. Mucus is mainly a water-based mixture of many secretions and exfoliated epithelial cells, but its exact makeup changes all the time. Its other components contribute to its physical and functional properties, such as mucins, which are large glycoproteins. Along the length of the gastrointestinal tract, the mucous layer varies in thickness. This mucous layer is continuous in organs such as the stomach and duodenum whereas further down the gastrointestinal tract there may be areas where there is no mucus. Mucus is constantly debrided from the surface of the gastrointestinal tract by abrasion, acids and enzymes, and resupplied from below over a few hours. The mucus is thicker in the stomach because it needs to have a sufficiently robust barrier against gastric acids. As an adverse effect, drugs such as non-steroidal anti-inflammatory drugs (**NSAID**s) and steroids can prevent the production of mucus of the appropriate constitution and consistency, which collectively compromise this protective barrier, resulting in damage to the gastric lining.

The gastrointestinal tract has several barriers that ensure that only the essential building blocks of life, such as glucose, amino acids and vitamins, are absorbed. This is a defence mechanism designed to mitigate the risk of **toxicity**. Of course, drugs are absorbed, so this is not a perfectly evolved system, but in summary, the barriers are as follows:

- pH and enzymes – many toxins are ionised at alkaline pH which corresponds to the pH of the small intestine, the site of maximum drug absorption
- Gastrointestinal mucosa
- Metabolic state prior to the onset of systemic disease

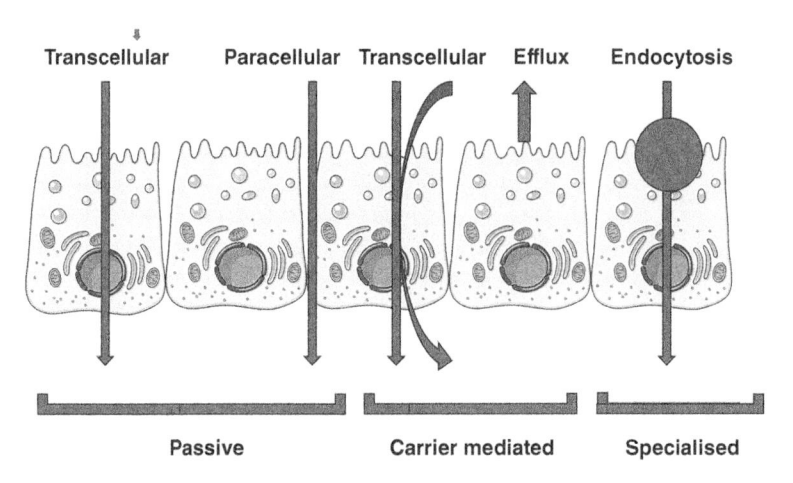

**Figure 2.3** Mechanisms of drug absorption

*Source*: Created using Servier Medical Art. Servier Medical Art is licenced under https://creativecommons.org/licenses/by/3.0/

The five mechanisms (described in Chapter 1; see Figure 2.3) by which drugs are absorbed through the gastrointestinal membrane are:

1. Transcellular
2. Paracellular
3. Active transport
4. Endocytosis
5. Passive or facilitated diffusion

To offer some examples, insulin and the cardiac glycoside group of drugs are transported by paracellular transport, vitamin B12 complex by active transport with **lipophilic** drugs (e.g. those which are required to enter the central nervous system and cross the blood–brain barrier by passive diffusion).

## Oesophagus

The mouth is the primary route of administration for most drugs. Contact with the oral mucosa is usually very short because patients tend to swallow quickly. The oesophagus connects the oral cavity to the stomach via the gastro-oesophageal junction. The oesophagus is made up of a thick muscular layer that measures approximately 250 millimetres in length and 20 millimetres in diameter.

Apart from the lower 20 mm, which resembles the gastric mucosa, the oesophagus is lined with a well differentiated squamous epithelium of non-proliferating cells. The oesophagus has glands that secrete mucus into the lumen to lubricate food and protect the lower part of the oesophagus from stomach acid. The oesophageal lumen typically has a pH of between 5 and 6. The act of swallowing transports materials down the oesophagus. Following ingestion, a single peristaltic contraction wave travels down the length of the oesophagus, increasing in speed. After the initial swallow, secondary contractions occur spontaneously to push any remaining sticky lumps of material or refluxed material into or back to the stomach. Gravity helps materials through the oesophagus when in the upright position. The oesophageal transit time for dosage forms is extremely short, typically between 10 and 14 seconds. Whilst the oesophagus does not play a role in drug absorption it can be affected by drugs. For example, the instruction to individuals prescribed doxycycline capsules, an antibacterial drug to take with a full glass of water, preferably in a standing or sitting position, is because doxycycline is caustic to the oesophagus. Because the mucus here is not as protective as that found in the stomach, there is a risk of ulceration if the drug becomes lodged.

## Stomach

The stomach is the next section of the gastrointestinal tract that food and pharmaceuticals will encounter. The stomach serves three primary functions.

1. A reservoir for ingested food to slowly deliver it to the duodenum to make sure the duodenum does not receive volumes too great for it to function optimally
2. Acid and enzyme digestion to make chyme which is a uniform creamy paste that helps absorption further down the gastrointestinal tract. It does this because the paste ensures greater contact between the ingested foods and the mucus membrane of the intestines than would blocks of food
3. Protection of the intestine by preventing toxins from reaching it. Drugs and toxins can be destroyed by the enzymes and acids in the stomach

The pyloric sphincter controls its connection to the duodenum. The stomach is anatomically divided into five regions (see Figure 2.4).

1. The cardia
2. The fundus
3. The corpus (body)
4. The antrum
5. The pylorus

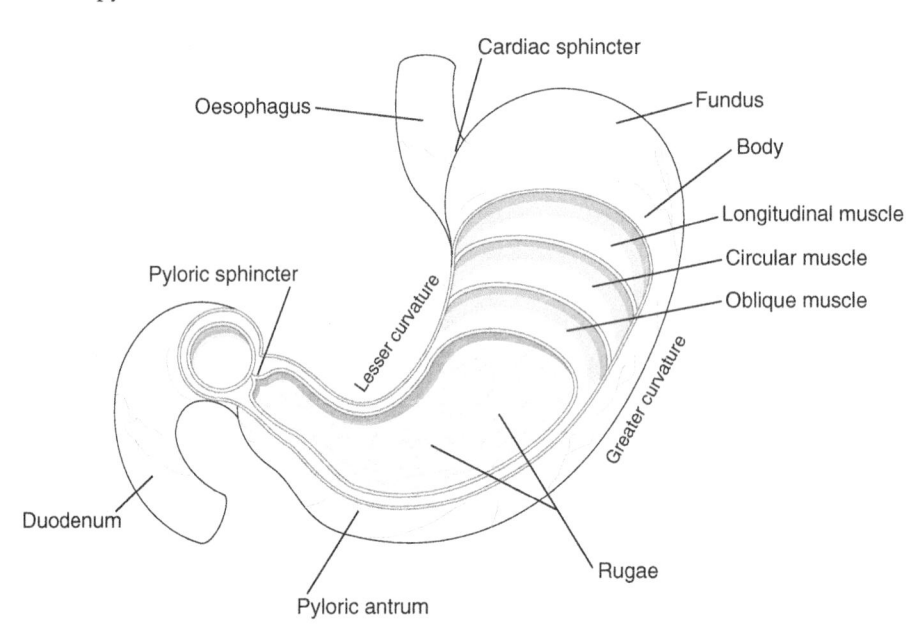

**Figure 2.4** The stomach

Although the stomach usually contains small amounts of fluid, often less than 50mL, it can hold about 1.5L if necessary.

The secretions of the stomach are:

- HCl secreted by parietal cells, maintaining the stomach's pH at 1–3.5 during fasting
- The hormone gastrin, that stimulates the gastric acid and pepsinogen production from the stomach's G cells. Gastrin is released in response to peptides, amino

acids and gastric distension, which results in increased gastric motility. Pepsins are peptidases that degrade proteins to peptides when the pH is low. Pepsin is denatured above pH 5
- Mucus, secreted by the mucous-neck cells that line the gastric mucosa. Mucus protects the gastric mucosa digesting itself with its own pepsin-acid combination. Without an effective mucous layer gastritis and ulceration can result

Surprisingly, the stomach absorbs very little medication because of its tiny surface area in comparison to the small intestine. In relation to medication, a factor for consideration is that the rate of gastric emptying determines how quickly drug absorption from the small intestine can start to happen. This is significant because the small intestine is where most drug absorption occurs.

The pH of the stomach is typically between 1 and 4. As a result, acidic drugs are largely non-ionised and can be absorbed through the stomach (e.g. aspirin). However, because the small intestine has a much larger absorptive surface area (even for acidic drugs), most absorption occurs there and not in the stomach.

Even when there is no specific interaction, the adaptive phase of gastric emptying, when a meal has just been consumed, causes hormones like cholecystokinin to be secreted and this retains food and drugs (if they happen to be there at the same time) for longer in the stomach. The foods that do this the most are fatty foods as they cause the most secretion of cholecystokinin. Whilst the total amount of drug absorption will not be affected, the time to a peak in the systemic circulation will be delayed and that could delay therapeutic effect.

It is important to remember that some drugs need to be taken with food. This can be to enhance their effect, or to prevent an adverse effect. An example is ascorbic acid (vitamin C) which increases the absorption of iron. As another example, a fatty meal increases the **bioavailability** and pharmacokinetic variability of the absorption of the antiretroviral saquinavir. It is uncertain why this is, but it could be because the drug becomes enveloped by lipid and absorbed within the lymphatic system, thereby avoiding first-pass metabolism.

---

### PAUSE AND REFLECT 2.1

Reflect on the impact of lifestyle factors on drug therapy. Think about a medication that requires dietary restrictions or lifestyle modifications. How do these factors influence the drug's effectiveness and safety?

---

## Intestine

The small intestine, the ileum, is the gastrointestinal tract's longest most complicated segment. It begins at the stomach's pyloric sphincter to the ileo-caecal junction and at that point meets up with the colon. It has a diameter of approximately 25 to 30 mm.

Its primary functions are:

- *Digestion*: The small intestine completes the process of enzymatic digestion that began in the stomach.
- *Absorption*: The small intestine is the site of greatest absorption from the gastrointestinal tract.

There are three parts to the small intestine: the duodenum, the jejunum and the ileum (see Figure 2.5).

The small intestinal wall is densely packed with blood and lymph vessels. This is the area of gastrointestinal tract with the best blood supply, which is crucial for absorption as this creates concentration gradients. In fact, the blood supply accounts for about 30% of total cardiac output via the superior mesenteric artery. The small intestinal circulation flows into the hepatic portal vein, which transports it to the systemic circulation via the liver. The liver metabolises drugs prior to them reaching the systemic circulation; this process is referred to as first-pass metabolism.

The small intestine wall also contains lacteals, which contain lymph and are therefore a component of the lymphatic system. The lymphatic system plays a critical role in fat absorption from the gastrointestinal tract; some drugs can be absorbed in this way and bypass **first-pass metabolism** after fatty meals.

The small intestinal surface area is significant and has adaptations that increase the surface area more than 500 times what it would be if it was a smooth cylinder. These adaptations are:

- Submucosal folds that wrap around the intestine in a circular fashion and are particularly developed in the duodenum and jejunum. They have a depth of several millimetres
- Villi, which are finger-like projections into the lumen (approximately 0.5–1.5 mm in length and 0.1 mm in diameter). They have an abundance of blood vessels. Each villus contains an arteriole, a venule and a lymphatic vessel that never ends (lacteal)
- Microvilli – 600–1000 of these brush-like structures with a length of 1um and a width of 0.1 um cover each villus, providing the greatest surface area increase

The small intestinal luminal pH increases to between 6 and 7.5. The secretions that produce these pH values in the small intestine come from the following sources:

- Brunner's glands, located in the duodenum, produce bicarbonate, which neutralises the acid excreted from the stomach.
- Intestinal flora are found throughout the small intestine and are responsible for the production of mucus and enzymes. The digestive process is continued by enzymes, hydrolases and proteases.

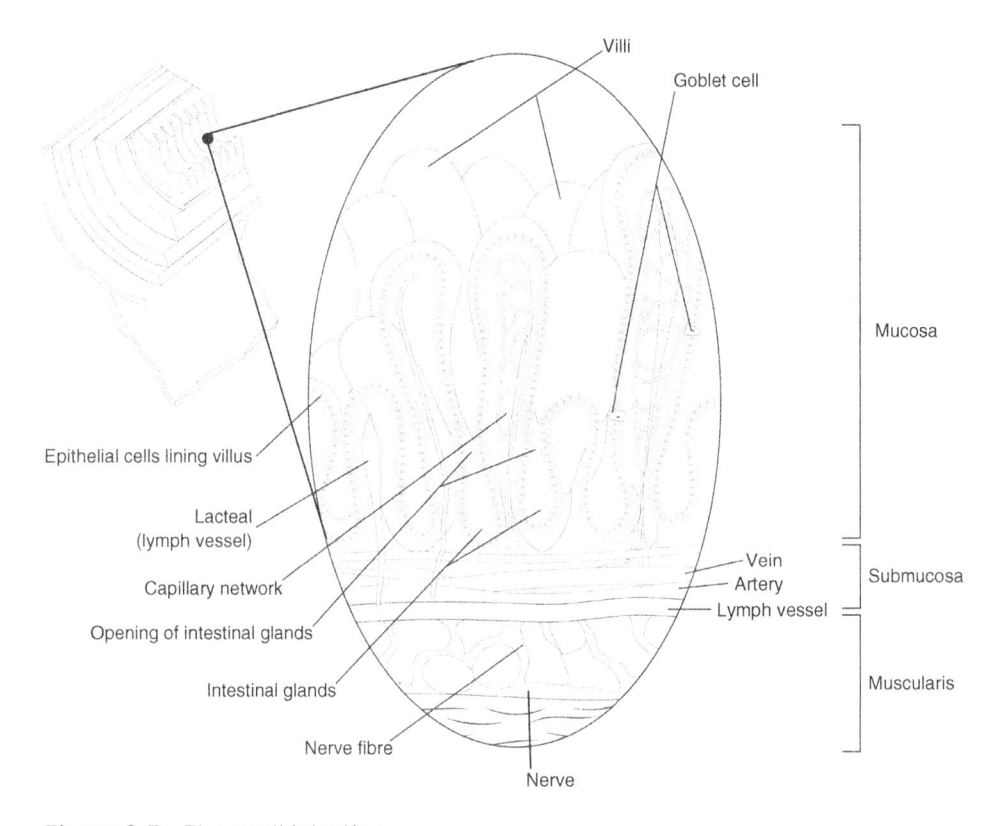

**Figure 2.5** The small intestine

- The pancreas secretes pancreatic fluid into the small intestine every day. Pancreatic juice is composed of sodium bicarbonate and proteases, lipase and amylase.
- Bile, a complicated mixture of organic and inorganic substances, is produced by the liver and stored in the gall bladder. It is made up of bile acids, phospholipids (especially lecithin, cholesterol, and bilirubin) as well as other organic and inorganic substances (such as the plasma electrolytes sodium and potassium). Bile pigments, the most common of which is bilirubin, are removed from the body in the faeces. Bile acids, on the other hand, are reabsorbed in the terminal ileum through a process that is very active as the body can reuse them. Because of their high clearance rate in the liver, they return to the liver through the portal vein and are then released into the bile again. The term 'enterohepatic recirculation' is used to describe this phenomenon and it can happen to some drugs as well. The main function of bile is to help the body absorb fats from food, like fatty acids and cholesterol, by emulsifying and dissolving them into micelles and emulsions. It also helps the body get rid of waste products that have been broken down.

Unless drugs are administered intravenously, they must pass through the phospholipid membranes before they reach the systemic circulation. Fat-soluble drugs (lipophilic) are more likely to be absorbed in the intestines because of the prevalence of villi and microvilli. Water-soluble (hydrophilic) drugs can be absorbed through special transport mechanisms or facilitated diffusion. Even if all the drug is absorbed by the intestinal epithelium, it can be transported back into the intestinal lumen or metabolised by the liver, so not all doses may get to the systemic circulation. This is referred to a pre-systemic or first-pass metabolism. The principle of first-pass metabolism will be explained more fully in Chapter 4.

The rate and extent of drug absorption depends on the physiochemical properties of the drug along with the physiological conditions of the gastrointestinal system. In practice, oral drug absorption typically only varies person to person with a clinically significant effect in a subset of patients with certain characteristics or with a limited number of drugs.

## PHYSIOLOGICAL FACTORS THAT INFLUENCE THE RATE AND EXTENT OF ABSORPTION

There are a number of physiological factors that influence the rate and extent of absorption, outlined in the next section of this chapter.

### Gut Motility and Transit Time

Gut transit time is defined as the time it takes for food to move through the gastrointestinal tract from the mouth to the anus, and will vary with age, sex, dietary habits or disease (see Figure 2.6 on gut motility). For example, if drugs move through the small intestine quickly (i.e. diarrhoea) then the contact time is reduced and hence the extent of absorption. This may be particularly problematic for modified-release drugs when absorption should take place over several hours. Alternatively, if drugs are held in the stomach for a long time before exiting, then absorption may be delayed. An example is metoclopramide, which increases the rate of gastric emptying and is therefore prescribed for nausea and vomiting.

### The Polarity of the Drug

Drugs defined as '**polar**' are highly water soluble. Polar drugs move poorly, or not at all, across cell membranes, which are mainly composed of lipids. Some drugs are so highly water soluble that they do not cross the cell membranes of the gut and cannot enter the systemic circulation. A good example of this is gentamicin which is so water soluble that it can only be delivered systemically by injection. This is a general rule, but it should be remembered that some polar molecules can cross cell membranes through specific transport mechanisms or channels. For example, glucose, a polar molecule, is absorbed

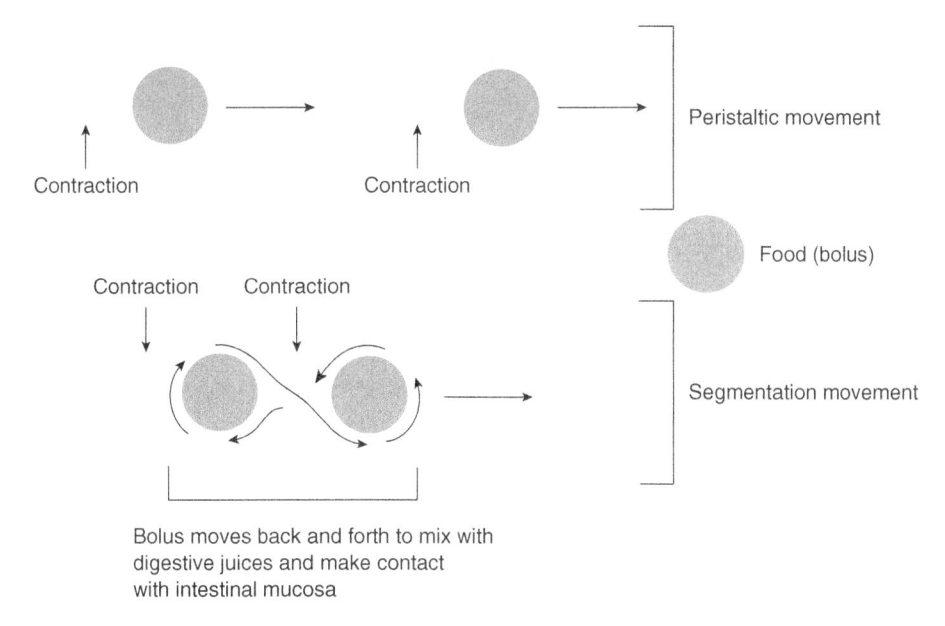

**Figure 2.6** Gut motility

in the small intestine primarily through a process called facilitated diffusion which is supported by specialised glucose transporter proteins embedded in the cell membranes of epithelial cells lining the small intestine.

## Changes to pH Within the Gastrointestinal Tract

The extent to which a drug is absorbed depends on the pH within the gastrointestinal tract. For example, aspirin is an acidic drug so is non-ionised (uncharged) in the stomach environment, which is itself acidic. Therefore the drug can cross cell membranes more easily. However, even though aspirin becomes ionised in the small intestine, the large surface area and good blood supply still means that most of the absorption of aspirin occurs here. Surface area and diffusion gradients surpass all other factors. Some drugs (e.g. **antacids**) and proton pump inhibitors will alter the pH of the stomach and may alter the extent of dissolution of the drug and subsequent extent of absorption. For example, whilst antacids (e.g. aluminium hydroxide) will increase the absorption of beta-blockers (e.g. propranolol), anti-fungal agents (e.g. ketoconazole) require this acidic environment for dissolution and therefore any drugs which increase the gastric pH will result in reduced absorption.

The presence of physiological enzymes can result in the destruction of some drugs which means they cannot be taken orally for a systemic effect. For example, peptide hormones such as insulin are denatured by gastric acid and digested by the gastrointestinal tract in the same way that proteins from our diet would be.

## Drug-Drug Interactions

The concomitant administration of drugs may result in variations in treatment failure or drug toxicity by affecting the extent and rate of drug absorption. This may be because there is a delay in the dissolution of the drug in the stomach, or gastric emptying and gut transit time are affected. Prokinetic agents prescribed to increase the rate of gastric emptying (e.g. metoclopramide for nausea and vomiting) risk increasing the rate of absorption of other drugs but in the case of digoxin, an increase in gut motility has the opposite effect. By reducing the contact time with the absorptive surface of the gastrointestinal tract, a reduction in the rate of absorption is seen. This is particularly noticeable with drugs administered as controlled-release or modified-release formulations. Alternatively, metoclopramide may increase the absorption of alcohol or paracetamol. Iron can reduce the absorption of the Parkinsonian drug, levodopa.

> ### PAUSE AND REFLECT 2.2
>
> Reflect on the concept of drug-drug interactions. Choose two or three commonly prescribed medications and investigate whether they have any known interactions. How do these interactions affect the efficacy or safety of the drugs involved?

## Drug-Food Interactions

The influence of food on drug absorption is highly complex and somewhat unpredictable (see Table 2.1). The presence or absence of food in the stomach may inhibit, enhance or delay drug absorption and hence affect the extent of drug availability. It is important to note that the specific effect can vary greatly depending on the drug. Some drugs are better absorbed with food, while others are absorbed more effectively on an empty stomach.

Some drugs are termed 'acid labile', which means they are susceptible to alteration in acidic environments. An example of this is flucloxacillin. Patients given the oral form of this drug are advised to take it an hour before food or a couple of hours after. This is because when we start eating, or are about to, our body lowers gastrointestinal pH ready for the meal to be eaten. This then would reduce the amount of flucloxacillin that could be absorbed and will result in treatment failure or **antimicrobial** resistance. Alternatively, if gastric pH is increased, for example if drugs such as proton pump inhibitors like omeprazole are taken (these treat gastro-oesophageal reflux disease, or stomach ulcers) then drugs like the anti-fungal itraconazole or the antiretroviral atazanavir are not absorbed to the same extent.

Tetracycline should not be administered with milk as it contains metal ions (e.g. calcium and magnesium) or drugs like antacids which contain aluminium salts.

The molecular complex which is formed (the process is commonly known as 'chelation') is too large to be absorbed and tetracycline will not have any therapeutic effect.

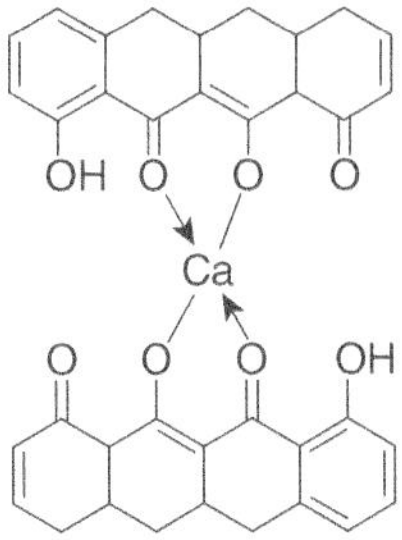

**Figure 2.7** An example of calcium chelation

Some foods affect absorption. In Figure 2.7 calcium from milk or antacids has bonded to two tetracycline molecules and now the structure is too large to be absorbed.

**Table 2.1** Levels of absorption in common drugs and food

| Drug | Food | Interaction |
| --- | --- | --- |
| Iron | Vitamin C | Increases absorption |
| Iron | Phytates – e.g. found in wholegrains, seeds and nuts | Decreases absorption |
|  | Tannin in tea | Decreases absorption |
| Tetracycline | Milk | Decreases absorption |
| Iron or tetracyclines | Calcium salts | Increases absorption |
| Levodopa | Protein-containing food | Decreases absorption |
| Albendazole (antiprotozoal agent) | Lipid-containing food | Increases absorption |

## Pathology Affecting the Jejunum and Ileum

The extensive surface area of the ileum allows for maximum drug absorption. However, several factors may affect both the rate and extent of absorption.

The functional integrity of the gastrointestinal tract will adversely influence absorption. For example, disease (e.g. Crohn's Disease), malabsorption syndrome or surgical resection will result in variability of the rate and extent of drug absorption. Malabsorption syndrome will reduce the absorption of drugs. Similarly intestinal obstruction will reduce peristalsis, drug movement through the gastrointestinal tract and drug absorption.

Coeliac disease risks reducing the surface area of the ileum, altering intestinal transit time and permeability of the gut wall which independently and collectively affect drug absorption.

## Age-Related Changes

In the older adult, a reduction in gastric hydrochloric acid production and pepsin, with a resultant decrease in gastric pH, may affect the solubility of drugs and hence the extent of absorption. Whilst these changes are not pharmacologically significant, the absorption of calcium drugs may be affected and there is a risk of early dissolution of enteric-coated drugs (e.g. aspirin, erythromycin) which may result in adverse gastric effects. A reduction in the active transport mechanisms may also affect the absorption of iron and vitamin B12, so if given as a treatment they may need to be given by a different route.

Similarly, a reduction in the blood flow to the intestinal wall and a loss in the number of absorbing cells collectively risk affecting absorption. Age-related reduction in gut motility will prolong the movement of the drug from the stomach to the small intestine. For drugs which are primarily absorbed in the upper small intestine (e.g. paracetamol), absorption will be delayed as will its pharmacological action.

## Reduction in Gut Motility in People Who Are Critically Ill

The rate and extent of oral absorption becomes unpredictable for many reasons in acute and critical illness. During physiological stress, the sympathetic nervous system is activated, which results in a decrease in the blood supply to the jejunum and ileum and a resultant increase in cardiac, renal and hepatic supply. This will have an adverse effect on the extent of drug absorption and is likely to cause enteral feed intolerance.

The use of supplementary feeding regimes via nasogastric tubes, percutaneous endoscopic gastrostomy or jejunal devices can result in absorption problems due to drug interaction with enteral feeds. For example, the bioavailability of phenytoin can be reduced as can the antimicrobial ciprofloxacin.

## Presence of Drug-Metabolising Enzymes in the Gut

The small intestine is a potential site for drug metabolism. The concept of drug metabolism is more fully explored in Chapter 4 but suffice to say that the presence of enzymes in the intestinal epithelial cells results in extrahepatic metabolism of several drugs (e.g. ciclosporin, nifedipine and verapamil). Grapefruit juice has been shown to inhibit the action of the CYP3A cytochrome 450 isoenzyme, a drug-metabolising enzyme found in the liver and intestine, and will therefore increase the availability of felodipine, for example.

## Dissolution of Drugs by Digestive Enzymes or Activity of the Gut Flora

Chloramphenicol, an antimicrobial agent, is degraded by gut microbes, reducing its bioavailability, whilst for several drugs (e.g. digoxin and steroid hormones) bioavailability is enhanced.

## Physical and Chemical Properties of the Drug

The extent and rate of drug absorption can be purposefully influenced by the formulation of the drug. Before absorption can take place, a tablet or capsule must be dissolved or disintegrated, whereas liquids will be absorbed faster. Tablets can be coated or uncoated. It may simply be that a sugar coating is more palatable, or the drug preparation is designed not to release in the stomach but in the small intestine (e.g. bisacodyl can irritate the stomach and induce nausea and enteric-coated erythromycin improves bioavailability as it is destroyed by gastric acids). However, it is important to note that enteric-coated aspirin and prednisolone cannot prevent the systemic effects of these drugs on the stomach, which may far outweigh the local irritation.

Some enteric coatings are developed to deliver the drug to a specific site within the gastrointestinal tract, for example sulfasalazine in the treatment of Crohn's disease needs to be further down in the gastrointestinal tract rather than in the acidic stomach or the alkaline small intestine.

This highlights the reason to avoid crushing enteric-coated tablets since this might result in medicines being released prematurely, to be destroyed by stomach acid, or to irritate the stomach lining.

Extended-release products are designed to release drugs over a longer period, typically 12 to 24 hours. This may be advantageous to avoid frequent dosing of the drug or to avoid the short-term side effects seen with high plasma concentrations. Whilst extended-release formulations are designed to create a constant plasma drug concentration, it is still worth remembering that there will still be minor fluctuations during drug release. Extended-release formulations usually have abbreviations on the drug packs such as CR (controlled release), ER (extended release), MR (modified release) to SR (sustained release), but other abbreviations exist. The way that the extended release is achieved varies significantly from coating the tablets in a slowly dissolving polymer, to embedding them in a matrix like MST Continus, or even to just making the particle size of the drug larger or the form more insoluble as in Tegretol Retard and Adalat Retard. In cases where the gut transit time is increased (e.g. diarrhoea) there will be a reduction in drug absorption.

It is extremely important not to change the formulation of the drug by crushing an extended-release formulation as this will alter the extent of absorption. It is likely to result in an unintentional and hazardous bolus dose that could cause an overdose.

In summary, the factors which affect the dissolution and absorption of a drug from the form administered, the drug's solubility and the ability of the drug to effectively traverse the small intestine to enter the mesenteric vessels and ultimately the systemic circulation as a therapeutic dose are summarised in the list below:

- The formulation of the drug
- Drug-drug interactions
- Drug-food interactions

- Gastric pH
- Integrity of the gastrointestinal tract
- Gastric motility
- Gastric emptying time
- Intestinal transit time and motility
- Length and vascularity of the gastrointestinal tract
- Expression of intestinal metabolising enzymes
- Intestinal pH
- Enterohepatic recycling

## Colon

The colon is the gastrointestinal tract's final organ. It goes from the ileo-caecal junction to the anus and makes up about 25% of the length of the gastrointestinal tract. It comprises the ascending, descending and sigmoid colon, and the rectum (see Figure 2.8).

Whilst the ileum has specialised villi, the colon does not. However, there are crypts in the colon, and there are irregularly folded mucosae. All these things make the colon's surface area ten times bigger than a simple cylinder, but this is still 30 times less surface area in comparison to the ileum. Therefore, the colon is not a major area of drug absorption.

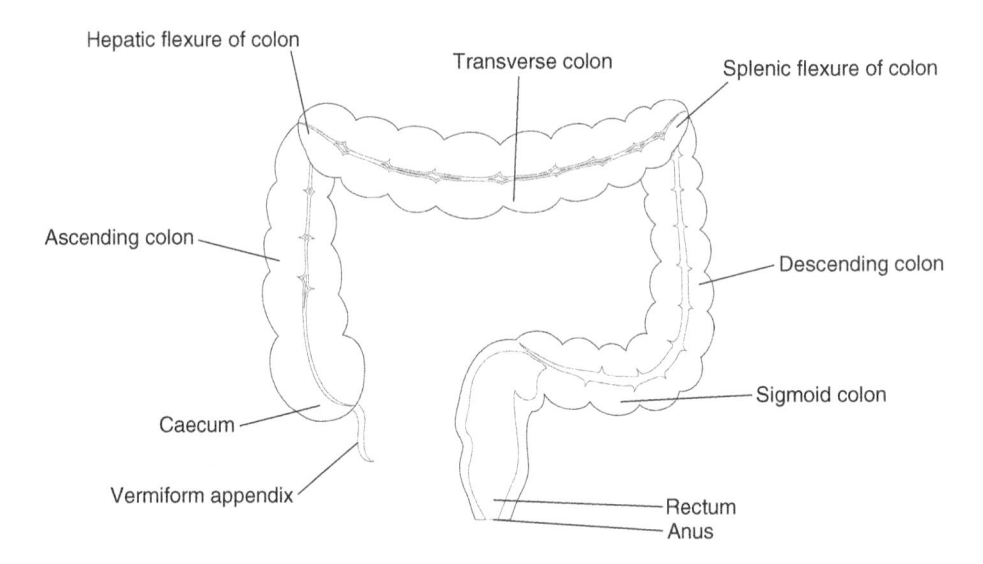

**Figure 2.8** Anatomy of the colon

The colon's primary functions are:

- Absorption of water and electrolytes
- Storage and compaction of faeces
- Maintenance of gut microbiota

The colon is permanently colonised by a diverse array of bacteria. This massive bacterial population is capable of a variety of metabolic reactions, including the breakdown of fats and polysaccharides. The bacteria rely on undigested polysaccharides and carbohydrates from secretions such as mucus for their energy. The caecum's pH ranges between 6 and 6.5 rising to 7 to 7.5 in the distal colon. Affecting the bacterial flora can have several effects relating to drug absorption. For example, some metabolised drugs can be excreted in bile. The bacteria in the gastrointestinal tract then metabolise these conjugated drugs back to their active form and they can be reabsorbed. Antibiotics that change the bacterial composition of the gut might then affect this system and reduce the amount of drug that is absorbed back into the systemic circulation within the colon. For example, oral antibiotics are thought to reduce the effectiveness of certain oral contraceptives. The antibiotics may destroy the bacteria in the gut that deconjugate the contraceptive and prevent it being reabsorbed. This puts women who take these oral contraceptives at the same time as antibiotics at risk of contraceptive failure.

### Rectum

The extent of drug absorption from the rectum is variable and this, along with patient preference, limits it adoption. However, the rectum is used to administer drugs either for a local effect (e.g. laxatives, steroids) or when the oral route is not suitable (such as benzodiazepines during seizure activity). One of the complicating factors is that drugs absorbed from the upper part of the rectum will be transported to the liver and undergo first-pass metabolism, whilst drugs absorbed from the lower part of the rectum will enter systemic circulation directly. The conventional thinking is that, in general, 50% of the drug that is absorbed from the rectum will avoid the first-pass effect.

The challenge is determining where the upper part of the rectum ends and the lower part begins during conventional administration of suppositories or other rectal medicines. Similarly, there are differences in the anatomy of individuals' venous drainage from the rectum that will also affect absorption, poor venous drainage leading to decreased absorption. Conditions that can affect the integrity of the rectal barrier such as anal fissures and ruptured haemorrhoids can lead to increased drug absorption.

## ENTERAL DRUG ADMINISTRATION

The following section introduces you to several pharmacological concepts which relate to the enteral route of drug administration.

### First-Pass Metabolism (Pre-Systemic Metabolism)

When an orally administered drug is absorbed from the lumen of the small intestine of the gastrointestinal tract (GIT), it enters the mesenteric vessels which in turn join to form the large hepatic portal vein. This blood is rich in absorbed nutrients as well as drug molecules. The hepatic portal vein takes this nutrient-rich blood to the liver. However, one of the main roles of the liver is detoxification, which includes drug metabolism, and so, to a greater or lesser extent, some of the drug dosage which has been absorbed may be destroyed before it leaves the liver and enters the systemic circulation by the hepatic vein. This reduces the concentration of the active drug before it reaches its site of action. The presence of gut-metabolising enzymes can also result in a reduction in active drug availability. This process is called first-pass metabolism. When a drug is developed, the drug's 'bioavailability' or 'oral availability' is published as part of the drug's pharmacokinetic profile. This represents the percentage of the originally administered drug which leaves the liver. Several drugs undergo significant first-pass metabolism that means they cannot be administered orally but other routes must be employed (e.g. intravenous administration) where drugs have 100% bioavailability as they bypass first-pass metabolism (see Figure 2.9).

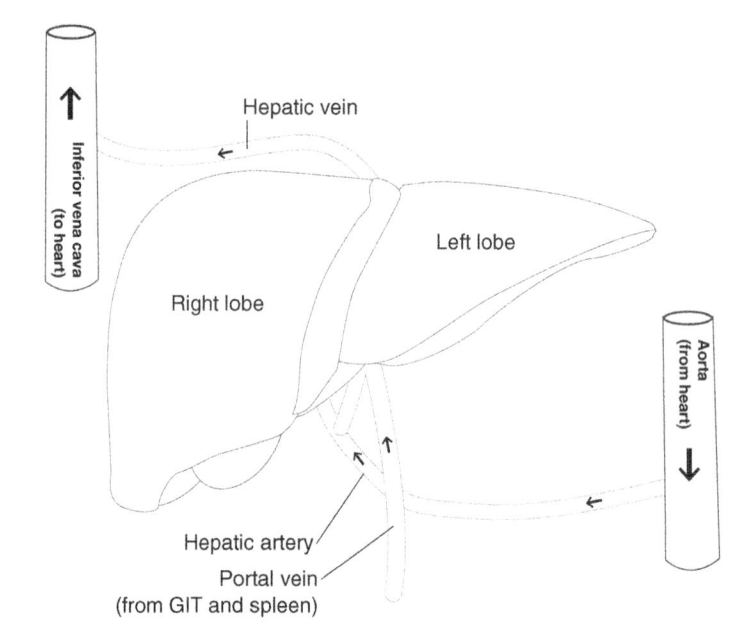

**Figure 2.9** First-pass metabolism

Some drugs are significantly metabolised during first-pass metabolism. Morphine sulphate has 23% bioavailability and propranolol approximately 15%, which explains the significant differences in oral and IV doses for both these drugs.

## Bioavailability

The term 'bioavailability' describes the extent to which a substance is absorbed into the systemic circulation. It does not consider the rate of drug absorption but simply the extent. Bioavailability is expressed as a percentage of the systemic dose for intravenous administration of the drug which is 100%. A bioavailability of 0% indicates that no drug enters the systemic circulation, whereas 100% bioavailability indicates that the entire dose is absorbed into the systemic circulation. In hepatic failure, drugs may not be metabolised correctly and so may accumulate if dosing continues, as there is no way for the body to inactivate them. Prodrugs (e.g. ramipril for hypertension), are inactive forms of a drug made into pharmacologically active compounds once they have undergone first-pass metabolism in the liver. They can be developed for several reasons. Primarily their development is to improve the bioavailability of the active drug, getting more of it into the systemic circulation.

There are many differences in drug bioavailability and whilst it might be assumed that the same drug will have the same bioavailability, different pharmaceutical formulations, age, presence or absence of gastrointestinal disease and other medications all influence the percentage bioavailability (see Table 2.2). These factors undoubtedly influence the therapeutic dose achieved and may risk therapeutic failure or toxicity.

Some drugs are so extensively metabolised following first-pass metabolism that they cannot be administered orally (e.g. glyceryl trinitrate, streptomycin and gentamicin). Glyceryl trinitrate is metabolised to the extent that if swallowed rather than used sublingually very little or no glyceryl trinitrate will enter systemic circulation and the drug will have no effect. This resulted in the production of other drugs such as isosorbide mononitrate which could be taken orally as it was less subject to first-pass metabolism.

**Table 2.2** Drugs and bioavailability

| Drug – oral administration | % Bioavailability (oral availability) |
|---|---|
| atenolol | 56 |
| diazepam | 100 |
| digoxin | 70 |
| fluoxetine | 60 |
| lithium | 100 |
| nifedipine | 50 |

Different pharmaceutical formulations of the same drug can also affect the bioavailability such that there is potential for drug doses and effects to vary between formulations. The rate at which the drug is absorbed is also important (along with the extent of absorption), and this affects how long it takes to reach the peak plasma concentration. Slow-release drugs are sometimes used to make it easier to take the drug once a day or to avoid the short-term side effects that come with high plasma concentrations. People who want to use one of these preparations instead of the other may need to stay on the same brand unless the alternative brands are what is called 'bioequivalent'. This isn't the case for all modified release preparations but can be significant, especially in cases where small variations can have a big effect. As examples, drugs that are modified release and have a narrow **therapeutic window**, such as theophylline preparations, would be prescribed by brand to avoid inadvertent small variations in blood plasma levels that would result in toxic or sub-therapeutic drug levels.

> ### PAUSE AND REFLECT 2.3
>
> Identify the advantages, disadvantages and considerations when administering drugs via the enteral route.

### Buccal and Sublingual Routes (Oral Transmucosal)

These routes involve administering drugs using the oral cavity (mouth). Sublingual administration of a drug is the placing a drug under the tongue whilst buccal administration refers to placing the drug between the gums and cheek. They come in the form of tablets, films or sprays (see Figure 2.10).

Like topical medication, buccal and sublingual medication are transported via paracellular and transcellular routes (see next section). However, unlike topical medication drugs administered via the buccal and sublingual routes are designed to act systemically.

The buccal and sublingual mucosa comprise a layer of stratified squamous epithelium on the surface which is linked to underlying connective tissue (lamina propria and submucosa) by a basal lamina. Within this connective tissue, there is a network of blood capillaries where drugs that have permeated through the epithelium can enter the systemic circulation.

Just like the other routes mentioned above (i.e. transdermal, subcutaneous, intravenous), they can be good alternatives to the oral route for drug delivery, particularly for drugs that may be extensively metabolised due to the first-pass effect or that are susceptible to degradation within the gastrointestinal tract. For example, as discussed above, glyceryl trinitrate (or nitroglycerin) (GTN), a drug used in the treatment of angina, when administered orally is extensively metabolised due to the first-pass effect, and therefore is given by the sublingual route. Here it is well absorbed and rapidly taken up into the circulation. Buccal administration has a similar effect, and this route is used for more prolonged action over a few hours. This is because the sublingual mucosa has a thinner epithelium than the buccal mucosa.

These routes have further advantages. The mouth has a large area for drug application and is more easily accessible than other mucosa such as that found in the nose, rectum and vagina. The oral mucosa is more permeable and has higher **perfusion** than the skin, leading to the drugs being absorbed more readily. This is particularly

**Figure 2.10** The buccal and sublingual mucosa

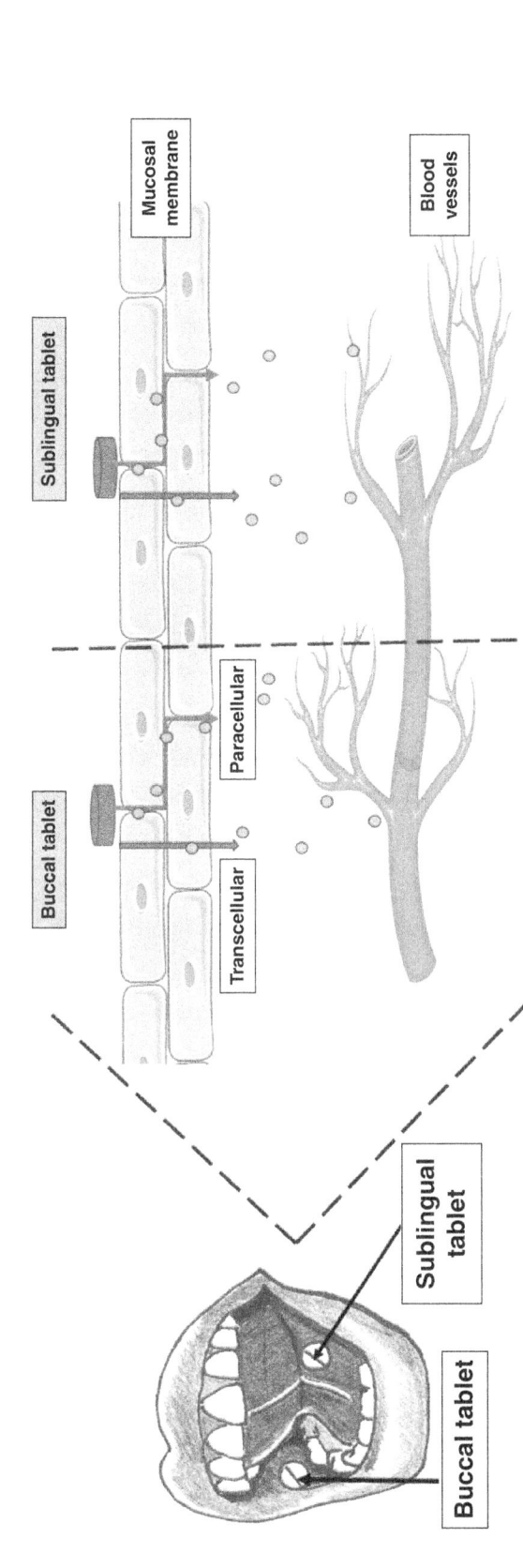

Source: Created using Servier Medical Art. Servier Medical Art is licenced under a Creative Commons Attribution 3.0 Unported License https://creativecommons.org/licenses/by/3.0/

important for drugs that need to be absorbed quickly such as GTN. When an individual is experiencing angina, GTN needs to be absorbed in a fast acting, easy and accessible way. The drug can quickly enter the systemic circulation, act upon vascular smooth muscle, causing it to relax and dilate, increasing blood flow to the heart and thus reducing the risk of myocardial infarction. Midazolam is another drug that requires a fast-acting approach. It is a benzodiazepine, used in reducing the length of seizures and in preventing early seizure recurrence. It can be administered via the buccal/sublingual route providing a more effective and socially acceptable alternative to the rectal route.

## TOPICAL AND TRANSDERMAL ADMINISTRATION

Topical and transdermal drugs are both applied to the skin. To understand the absorption of drugs via these methods it is important to have knowledge of the structures and functions of the skin.

### The Skin

The skin is the most accessible organ of the body. It is also the largest organ, covering a surface area of 1.7m² of the body, and the heaviest, weighing between 3.5 and 10 kgs, almost 16% of the total body mass of an individual. The skin is part of the integumentary system along with accessory structures such as hair, nails, oil glands and sweat glands and

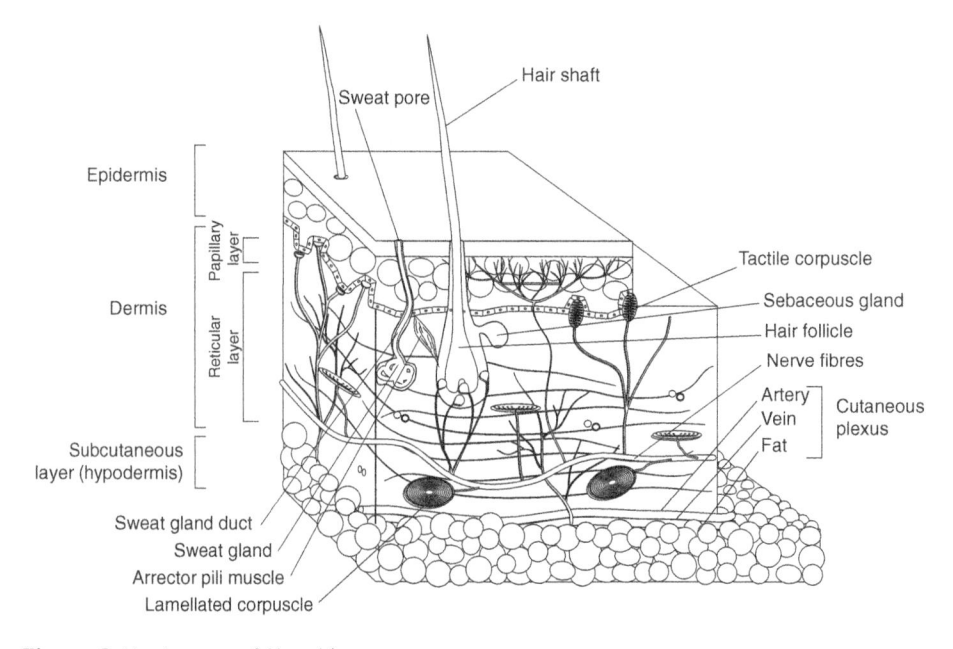

**Figure 2.11** Layers of the skin

their ducts. It has several functions, mainly to act as a protective barrier between the body and the external environment. This includes protection from the sun, micro-organisms, allergens, chemicals and loss of water. It comprises three layers: epidermis (the outermost layer), the dermis (the middle layer) and the hypodermis (the innermost layer also known as the subcutaneous layer). Let's explore these layers in more detail (see Figure 2.11).

## Epidermis

The epidermis comprises five separate layers, from the stratum germinativum (the innermost layer or basal layer which is attached to the dermis) to the outermost layer, the stratum corneum. It varies in thickness ranging from 0.5 mm on your eyelids to 4.0 mm on the heels of your feet. It consists mainly of keratinocytes but also contains melanocytes (which produce melanin and protect the skin from UV radiation), Langerhans cells (integral to providing an appropriate immune response to the environment they encounter) and Merkel cells (mechanoreceptors that are involved in the sensation of touch). The basal layer contains cuboidal, highly active epithelial cells which are constantly dividing. As new cells form, they are pushed up through the layers away from the nutrient and blood source located in the dermis. Their structure and shape change as they make this journey. Once they reach the outer layer the cells are dead, flat and thin in shape and mainly contain the fibrous protein keratin. They are known as corneocytes.

## Dermis

This layer is tough but elastic. It consists of collagen, connective tissues and elastic fibres. Blood vessels are located in the dermis, providing nutrients for both the dermis and the epidermis. It also contains sweat glands (and ducts), sebaceous glands and nerve endings. These nerve endings are specialised to detect touch, temperature, pressure and pain. The presence of these nerve endings means that the skin is one of the most important sensory organs in the body.

## Hypodermis

This is the deepest, innermost layer of the skin and is often called the subcutaneous layer. This acts as a contact layer between the skin and the underlying bones, muscle and tissue. The hypodermis mainly consists of fat cells, fibroblasts and macrophages and its main function is storage of energy and protecting the body from heat loss and harm. This will be explored in more depth later in administration by subcutaneous injection.

## Topical Delivery

A topical medication is one that is applied to a location on the body with the intention that it treats the condition or ailment locally or at the site of application. Topical medications are applied to mucous membranes (including those found in ears, eyes and the nose) but most often they are applied to the skin.

A transdermal medication is one whose use is intended to penetrate the skin and have a therapeutic effect on the tissues below and vessels below, often to have a systemic effect (see Figure 2.12).

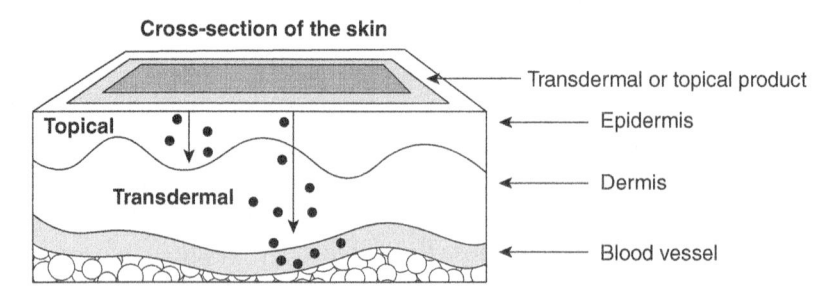

**Figure 2.12** A transdermal medication

Topical drug delivery can avoid the need for systemic administration of drugs, most commonly through the oral route. As it is acting directly at the site of delivery it can reduce the total drug dose needed and therefore the risk of adverse side effects.

Topical medications will contain materials both active (the drug) and inactive (the vehicle). The choice of vehicle will depend on where the drug is to be applied, how easy it is to apply, how long it remains on the skin and how it looks. The vehicle determines the consistency of the product which could be thick and greasy such as ointments, creams or gels or could be more watery such as lotions, foams or sprays. Ointments are generally better at delivering the active ingredient than creams because they are often more evenly applied and spread across the skin. However, creams are more easily absorbed, able to cover larger areas of skin and are also more readily accepted by individuals as ointments can be messy, greasy and difficult to wash off.

Topical delivery of drugs is predominantly used in the treatment of dry itchy skin, skin inflammation, allergic reactions and microbial and fungal infections.

One of the most common topical preparations used in the management of dry and itchy skin is emollient. **Emollients** moisturise the skin by increasing the amount of water stored in the stratum corneum. As the skin becomes dry by losing moisture, the corneocytes become smaller and gaps begin to open between the cells, which may reduce the barrier function of the epidermis. When applied to the skin, the emollient traps the water and rehydrates the corneocytes and mimics the natural lipid complex. The 'greasier' the substance the better the sealing and trapping of the water, such as those which have high concentrations of petroleum jelly. Some emollients also draw water from the dermis to the epidermis as they may contain substances known as humectants (e.g. urea and glycerine). Emollients are often used to manage skin conditions such as eczema. It is recommended that emollients are used as adjuncts to other therapies, such as topical/oral **corticosteroids** in the control of such chronic skin conditions. Some research suggests that emollients should be applied first, before topical corticosteroids, as this allows for the stratum corneum to be well hydrated and thus makes it easier for the corticosteroid to be absorbed, and that time should be left between applications, so the emollient does not to dilute the effects of the corticosteroid. National Institute for Health and Care Excellence (NICE, 2024) guidelines support this and recommend a 30-minute interval if practically possible.

For microbial and fungal infections of the skin, topical antibiotics and topical antifungals may be applied (e.g. erythromycin which is frequently used for the treatment of acne). Acne can be a chronic condition, starting in puberty and extending into adulthood. It is caused by the enlargement of the sebaceous glands and an increase in sebum production that is stimulated by the beginning of puberty. Also, an accumulation of keratin within the intrafollicular duct leads to a build-up of this sebum. These actions lead to the plugging of the hair follicles trapping *Cutibacterium acnes* (*C. acnes*) which ordinarily is a common and harmless bacterium, but thrives on the extra sebum, overgrows and produces an inflammatory response leading to skin lesions. Topical antibiotics such as erythromycin inhibit the enzyme and protein synthesis involved in bacterial growth. Due to the concern about the rise of antibiotic resistance over recent decades, topical antibiotics for acne are usually prescribed with another topical agent to reduce the length of time the antibiotics are required. The most common of these is benzoyl peroxide. This can help with the breakdown of keratin, therefore unblocking the drainage of sebum and 'unclogging pores', and also inhibiting the growth of *C. acnes*.

## Transdermal

Drugs administered transdermally are designed to penetrate the epidermis and dermis without accumulation in the dermal layer, to reach the deeper tissues and blood vessels beneath, thus having a systemic effect. This mode of absorption has several advantages over other routes. It avoids the first-pass effect and so increases the bioavailability of the drug. It can be an alternative to parenteral administration which can be painful and have a higher risk of infection. Transdermal routes benefit patients who are nil by mouth or who cannot swallow. It can also help with patient concordance, due to a reduction in dosage frequency. Furthermore, it has been found to administer the drug constantly and reliably, maintaining therapeutic blood levels and thus minimising side effects.

In order for the drug to reach the systemic circulation it must be able to permeate the dermis and the epidermis. The main barrier to this is the stratum corneum (this is also the case for topical medication).

The stratum corneum can be likened to a wall, with the corneocytes as the bricks and the intercellular lipid matrix being the cement or mortar. This construction is critical to its barrier function. If a drug formulation is applied to the skin surface it can cross the epidermis in three ways, through the (a) transappendegeal route, (b) the intracellular (transcellular) route or (c) the intercellular (paracellular) route. The route will depend on the chemical properties of the permeating drug molecule. Lipophilic or non-polar solutes will be mainly transported through the intercellular route (through the matrix layers) whilst hydrophilic or polar solutes will permeate via the intracellular route (through the corneocytes). The transappendegeal route allows drug molecules to move through the sweat glands and across hair follicles.

At present, most transdermal drugs have been delivered by adhesive patches. The patch increases drug absorption due to the longer application time. The drug is contained in high doses in a liquid or gel-based reservoir, which along with the occlusive nature of the patch drives the drug via passive diffusion through the skin. However, the drug must possess the right properties to passively permeate the skin (i.e. being lipophilic and of low molecular weight) and this often limits the variety of drugs that can be delivered transdermally. Chemical enhancers are often added to the medication to improve permeability by modifying the chemical barrier properties of the stratum corneum. The enhancers work in a variety of ways, including disruption of intercellular lipids, increase in the fluidity of the stratum corneum lipid bilayers and increase in thermodynamic activity. Some examples of chemical enhancers are alcohols, sulphoxides essential oils, fatty acids and urea. However, they can often cause skin irritation. There are many drugs that can be delivered transdermally (e.g. fentanyl, which is a strong **opioid** used to relieve chronic pain). Another common drug that uses patches for transdermal delivery is hyoscine. This is administered to prevent motion sickness and is placed on the postauricular area (the hairless area behind the ear) because the stratum corneum is at its thinnest in this location and therefore the drug is more readily absorbed.

Today, there are more 'active' transdermal delivery systems available that use non- and minimally invasive technologies, such as iontophoresis, microneedles, electroporation and sonophoresis, to enhance drug delivery across the skin and thus broaden the number of drugs that can be delivered transdermally. Iontophoresis and electroporation are both techniques that use electrical impulses to help deliver medication across the skin, whilst sonophoresis uses ultrasound to reduce the skins resistance. More recently, there has been intensive research into the use of microneedles. Patches support multiple microscopic projections or needles that are of a shape and length to avoid nerve endings in the dermis. One of the most favoured uses of this technique is for vaccinations, as they offer a pain-free method that could possibly be self-administered.

Transdermal patches are increasingly being used with children and young people and some have been particularly designed for use in children such as the methylphenidate patch for the treatment of attention deficit hyperactivity disorder. However, despite the advantages of this non-invasive and acceptable route of drug delivery for children and young people there are still issues with formulation for neonates who have an immature skin barrier. However, it is important to note that the extrauterine environment triggers rapid maturation, so that by two or three weeks of age the skin has similar barrier properties to that of a term infant.

In fact, age must be considered when administering topical/transdermal medication as the skin changes throughout the life stages of an individual. Young children have a thinner stratum corneum and larger skin-surface to body-mass ratio. Any topical drug is therefore likely to be absorbed much more readily than in an older child or adult due to the increased permeability of the skin.

As an individual grows older there are significant changes to the skin in both function and structure. However, evidence has shown that in practice there are no significant differences in absorption of drugs from transdermal delivery systems (Kaestli et al., 2008). The need for dose adaptation in elderly individuals is often not due to the absorption of the drug through the skin but to what happens when the drug reaches the systemic system and concerns with age-related cardiovascular, cerebral, hepatic and/or renal compromise that cause pharmacokinetic and pharmacodynamic changes.

# PARENTERAL ROUTES OF DRUG ADMINISTRATION

'Parenteral' means any non-oral means of administration, but usually refers to injecting directly into the body and bypassing the skin and mucous membranes, 'par' meaning 'beyond' and 'enteral' relating to the intestines. Parenteral routes are almost perfect ways of administering drugs due to the high bioavailability and quick onset of action. In intravenous (IV) drug administration, all the dose reaches the systemic circulation and has an immediate physiological response. In contrast, subcutaneous (SC) and intramuscular (IM) administrations involve an absorption process from the injection site leading to a more delayed and slower response. This is due to the drug molecules having to diffuse across the interstitial space to reach the capillaries. However, absorption is still a lot quicker than via the enteral route.

Common means of parenteral administration of drugs include subcutaneous, intravenous and intramuscular methods, which will now be explored.

## Subcutaneous Injection

As previously stated, the subcutaneous layer (hypodermis) is the deepest layer of the skin. It is mainly made up of fatty molecules and drugs can be administered directly and deposited into this layer via subcutaneous injection.

Subcutaneous administration is often required when drugs are not compatible with oral delivery as they may be highly metabolised by the first-pass effect or are partially or fully destroyed by the gastric juices such as insulin.

Insulin is a naturally occurring hormone that is secreted by the pancreas and is involved in the control of blood glucose levels. In type 1 diabetes, **endogenous** insulin is either minimal or non-existent and therefore SC insulin is administered to replace this deficiency. Insulin cannot be administered orally due to its chemical properties. It is a very large molecule and highly polar. It has difficulty crossing the gastrointestinal epithelium therefore as it is too polar to diffuse through the cell membrane and too big to move between the cells. Also, insulin is a protein, and proteins are extensively metabolised by enzymes present in the stomach. Therefore, delivering insulin via an SC injection ensures that it reaches its target cells.

Complications associated with subcutaneous injections include infection, abscess formation and lipohypertrophy. Lipohypertrophy, the accumulation of fatty scar tissue, can be caused by repeated injections in the same area of the skin and will display unpredictable drug absorption. The rotation of injection sites is recommended for this reason.

There are four recommended sites to inject into the SC tissue even though subcutaneous tissue is quite easy to reach from all injection sites on the body surface. These four sites are chosen because of the depth of SC tissue (see Figure 2.13).

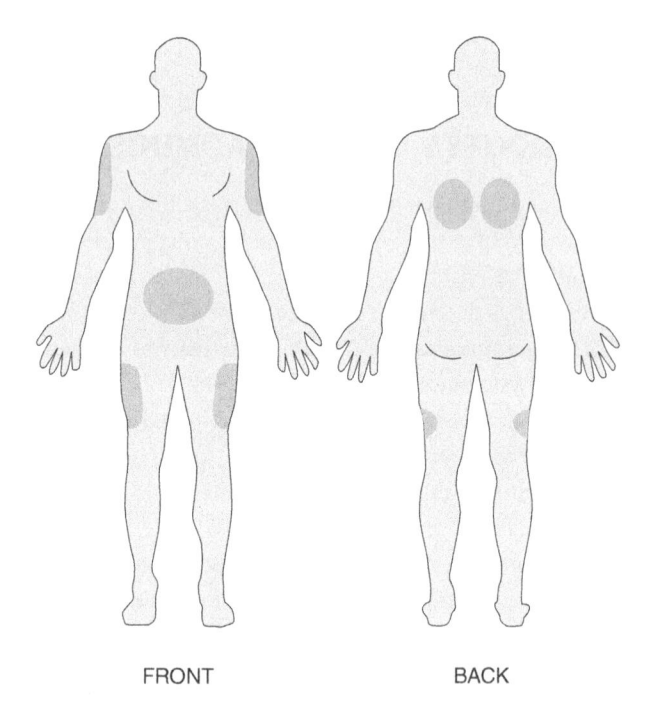

FRONT          BACK

**Figure 2.13** Four recommended sites for injection

*Source*: British Columbia Institute of Technology. http://open.bccampus.ca

Another example of a drug that is poorly absorbed in the gastrointestinal tract is heparin. This is due to its molecular size and ionic repulsion from negatively charged epithelial tissue in the gut and therefore has poor oral bioavailability. Heparin belongs to a family of **anticoagulant** drugs that activate the natural anticlotting protein antithrombin, which interrupts the factors involved in the clotting process of the blood. There are two forms of heparin in use which include original heparin and the more recent low-molecular-weight heparins such as tinzaparin, dalteparin and enoxaparin. These drugs are commonly given post-surgery where immobility may encourage clotting in the deeper veins of the legs.

Drugs administered subcutaneously are often small in volume, usually up to between 1.5 and 2 mls as larger volumes are associated with pain and adverse effects at the site. Subcutaneous administration is often used when drugs are required to be released more slowly (such as the examples above), because just as subcutaneous tissue can store fat, it can also provide a good depository for drugs that need to be absorbed gradually due to its limited blood flow.

There are several factors that may affect drug absorption via the SC route. including exercise and changes in environmental temperature. It is thought that the absorption of SC medications may increase during exercise because of increased blood flow to the area and the massaging effect of the exercising muscle. Conversely, drugs may not be absorbed so readily in patients with conditions where there is impaired blood flow, such as circulatory shock.

## Intramuscular Administration

Lying underneath the epidermis, dermis and subcutaneous tissue is skeletal muscle (see Figure 2.14). Skeletal (striated) muscle has an abundant blood supply and therefore the injected drug reaches the systemic circulation more quickly. Skeletal muscle can also absorb larger volumes of fluid due to the rapid uptake of the drug into the bloodstream via the muscle fibres. Due to this increase in drainage away from the muscle fibres, complications like abscess and granuloma formation are less common after intramuscular injections than after subcutaneous injections.

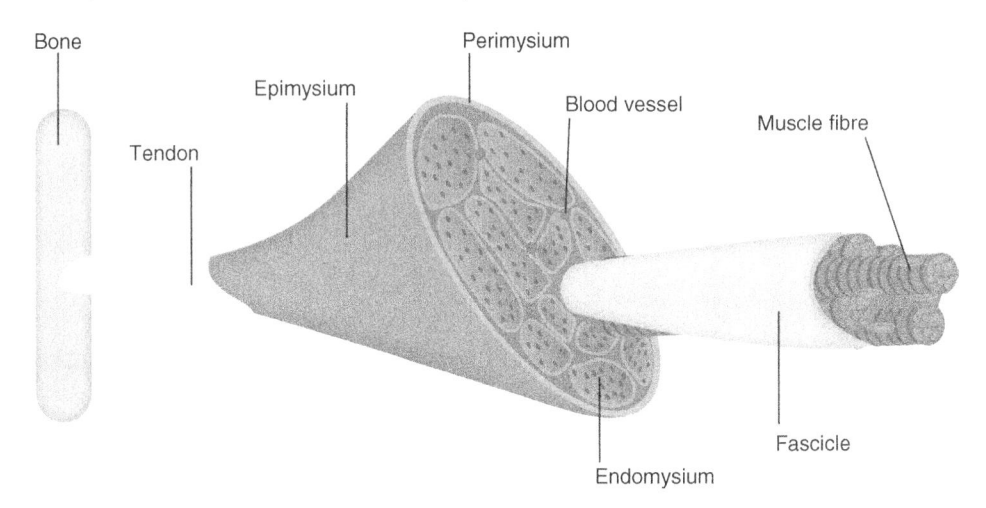

**Figure 2.14** Skeletal muscle

Also, the skeletal muscle contains fewer pain receptors than SC tissue and so IM injections can be less painful and can be utilised to deliver concentrated and irritant drugs that would otherwise damage the SC tissue.

There are a variety of recommended sites for IM injection which are often chosen because of patient preference and the volume of the drug that needs to be administered (see Figure 2.15). For smaller volumes (approximately up to 2 mls) the deltoid site can be used, whereas for larger volumes the ventrogluteal site is preferred in adults and the vasterus lateralis/rectus femoris in young infants. The ventrogluteal site is the site of choice as it is free of nerves and has a thick layer of muscle and a thin layer of fat, as opposed to the dorsogluteal site. Evidence suggests that using the dorsogluteal site comes with a high risk of administering the drug into subcutaneous tissue rather than the muscle and a high risk of damaging the sciatic nerve (Jung Kim and Hyun Park, 2014).

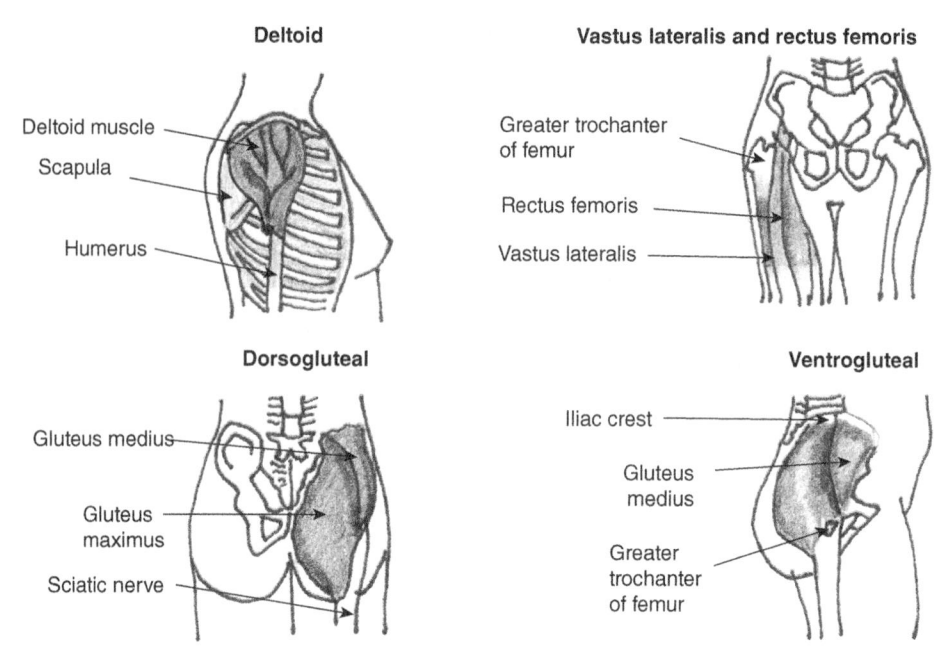

**Figure 2.15** Recommended sites for IM injection

IM injections are one of the most common procedures to be performed, although they are often avoided in children due to fear, pain and anxiety. However, there are also physiological and pharmacological reasons for not using the IM route in children. Young infants have less muscle mass and therefore absorption of the drug can be unreliable.

Ageing also brings about changes in body composition and older people have less muscle mass. This, along with reduced blood flow, leads to lower or unpredictable absorption of the drug.

Even though we try to avoid administering drugs to children via the IM route, some are routinely delivered this way, such as vaccinations. Most vaccinations are delivered via the IM route but there are some exceptions such as the BCG vaccine (for tuberculosis), which is delivered intradermally (just under the epidermis of the skin) and flu vaccine for children is delivered via nasal drops.

The IM route is chosen for a variety of reasons. Muscle contains many immune cells called dendritic cells that can recognise antigens and carry them to the lymph nodes. Lymph nodes act as reservoirs for white blood cells, which are a fundamental part of our immune response. The dendritic cell will present the antigen to the white blood cells causing them to multiply and start producing antibodies to defend our body against specific pathogens. The most common place for vaccines is in the deltoid muscle. This is close to the armpit which contains many lymph nodes and an abundance of white cells.

> **PAUSE AND REFLECT 2.4**
>
> Consider the advantages, disadvantages and other considerations when administering drugs via an intramuscular injection.

## Intravenous Route

Intravenous drug administration is the direct delivery of a drug into the venous, systemic circulation. The drug is administrated via devices (e.g. peripheral intravenous cannula, peripherally inserted central catheter (PICC), centrally inserted central catheter (CICC)) which are sited in the vein. As veins return deoxygenated blood via the inferior vena cava to the right side of the heart, the drug will be distributed around the body once it has passed through the cardiac chambers and into the aorta.

The administration of a drug directly into the venous, systemic circulation means that intravenous drugs are immediately available to the body for therapeutic action.

The advantages of intravenous drug administration include the following circumstances:

- Bioavailability is 100% as there are no barriers to absorption and the drug does not undergo first-pass metabolism
- There is minimal delay in drug response and it is therefore valuable in emergency situations (e.g. cardiac arrest)
- Drug titration – if a drug is administered via an intravenous infusion, then the dose can be manipulated to control the physiological response (e.g. blood glucose levels and insulin, noradrenaline infusion and blood pressure control, propofol (sedative) and sedation score)
- The infusion can be stopped if there are adverse effects. However, if the drug has a long **half-life**, then the drug effects will persist as they would with orally administered drugs (e.g. the drug amiodarone, prescribed for cardiac arrythmia, has a half-life of 50 days)
- Intravenously administered drugs with a relatively short duration of action (e.g. the sedative midazolam) are useful for invasive procedures where prolonged sedation is not required
- Administration of drugs which are poorly absorbed from the gastrointestinal tract, drug degradation by gastrointestinal enzymes or bioavailability is significantly compromised when administered orally and therefore they can only be administered intravenously (e.g. gentamicin)
- Several drugs administered via the intramuscular or subcutaneous route are painful because they risk staying in the muscle or adipose tissue respectively as a potential toxic concentration
- The intima of the vein is insensitive and therefore drugs which are irritating or non-isotonic can be administered
- Allows for the administration of large volumes of fluid

There are, however, several considerations and potential disadvantages to the intravenous administration of drugs, which include:

- Intravenous access devices are potential vehicles for microbial contamination, which risks the development of sepsis
- Risk of thrombophlebitis (e.g. diazepam), although improved drug formulations have reduced this risk
- Risk of necrosis caused by extravasation of the drug into the tissues. If the peripheral inserted cannula becomes displaced within the vein or the vein is ruptured during insertion of the access device, then the drug will enter the surrounding tissues and may lead to tissue death. This is seen particularly with **cytotoxic** drugs
- For drugs which are administered in intravenous fluids to dilute the drug prior to administration, there is a risk that the drug is incompatible with the **solvent/** dilution fluid. This incompatibility may result in precipitation of the drug out of solution and risk embolism. For example, drugs should not be administered to blood products: hypertonic mannitol results in the crenation (shrinkage and change in shape) of red blood cells; glucose results in the clumping of red blood cells
- Rapid drug delivery into the intravenous system may result in cardiac arrythmias or toxicity. For this reason, cardiac monitoring may be advised (e.g. phenytoin) or the drug is not licensed for IV administration (e.g. stemetil (anti-emetic))
- If the drug is administered too quickly, 'speed shock' is a systemic reaction resulting in flushing, headache and cardiac arrythmias
- Significant costs incurred due to consumables, personnel time and requirement for training and education

## INTRA-ARTERIAL DRUG ADMINISTRATION

The intra-arterial route involves the administration of the drug via an artery. This route is usually reserved for the administration of contrast medium for diagnostic purposes (e.g. angiography), direct delivery of the drug to treat neoplasms or the administration of vasodilators in arterial embolism (e.g. alteplase in ischaemic stroke).

The intra-arterial administration of drugs is contraindicated as an alternative route to intravenous administration as the drug would be delivered as a bolus directly to tissues, which would result in compromised tissue perfusion.

### Inhalation

The upper airway consists of the structures of the nose, nasal cavity, nasopharynx and oropharynx. The function of the upper airway is to provide initial protection to the internal environment of the body by warm filtering and humidifying the air entering

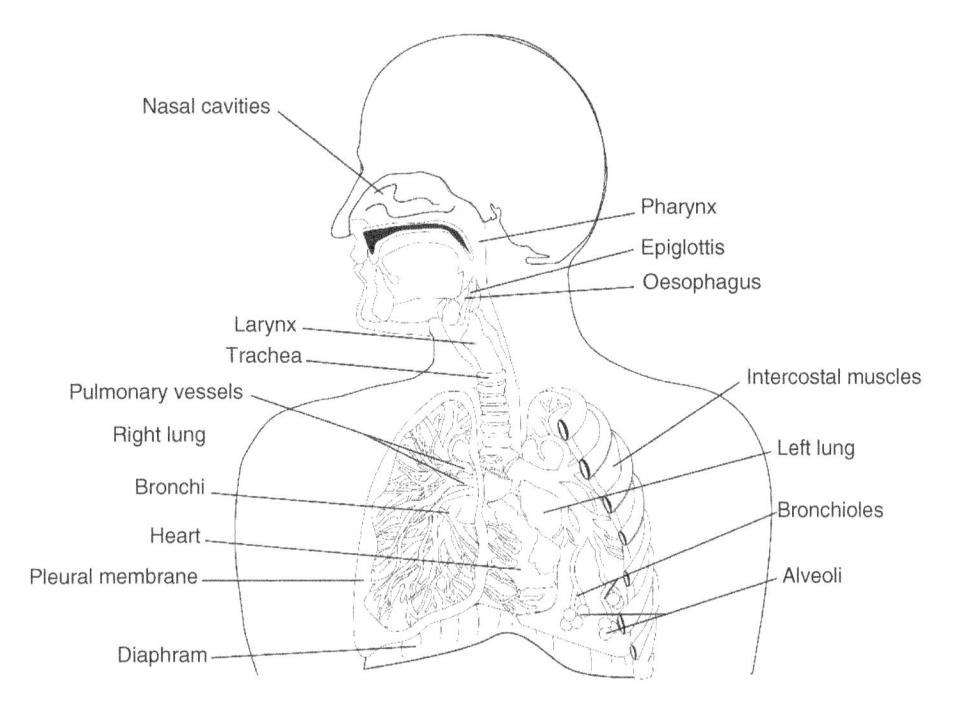

**Figure 2.16** Inhalation

the body. The folds of the nasal cavity provide an increased surface area with which to humidify and warm air entering the body to limit drying out of the lower airway and minimise insensible thermal loss. Small hairs in the nose and the mucous coating in the nasal cavity help capture and prevent larger airborne particles from progressing into the lower airway.

The lower airway consists of the larynx, trachea, left and right main bronchus, bronchi and bronchioles culminating in the alveoli. The trachea, bronchus and bronchi are predominantly surrounded by hyaline cartilage rings which serve to support the airway and help maintain its patency. It again has a layer of mucous which coats the internal lumen and helps capture any microparticulate debris that has managed to pass into the lower airway (see Figure 2.16).

The alveoli are the terminal point of this bronchial tree, and it is the site where gaseous exchange takes place, allowing oxygen to diffuse into the bloodstream and carbon dioxide out. This process of two-way **diffusion** is referred to as external respiration.

There are three distinct layers to a large proportion of the tissues within the respiratory tract: the uppermost layer (epithelium); the supportive structure below (lamina propria) is referred to commonly as the mucosa; below this exists the submucosa which contains the smooth muscle that envelops the airway and for the larger airway structures also contains cartilage. The final outer layer of the airway is the adventitia consisting primarily of connective tissue that anchors the structures within the organ system.

The large surface area of the pulmonary system, particularly the bronchial tree and alveoli spaces, are advantageous to drug delivery. Small-particle drugs (e.g. anaesthetic gases) are rapidly diffused across the alveolar membrane to induce effect, with bronchodilator therapies acting locally in the pulmonary structures. For drugs which are administered for local effect, the size of the drug particle is such that there is limited systemic absorption – for example, when administering salbutamol, a short-acting $\beta_2$ adrenergic receptor **agonist**, the systemic side effects of **tachycardia** and palpitations are reduced.

Drugs administered via the pulmonary system frequently adopt dry powder, aerosol pressurised metered-dose inhalers or nebuliser delivery systems. Developments in technology and design of devices have improved drug delivery; however, poor technique and user coordination will result in inconsistent drug deposition. Another factor to be considered is that pulmonary disease may be a barrier to successful drug delivery. The bronchoconstriction seen in asthma, airway obstruction by mucus plugging, hypersecretion or a foreign body will result in increased airway resistance. As the diameter of the airway reduces it becomes exponentially more difficult to pass the same volume of air through the respiratory tree, lowering the tidal volume, and therefore reducing the ability to transport any medication suspended within the air to the areas of the lung.

Reduced compliance is a reduction in the lung's elasticity and its ability to stretch. This can result from pneumonia, pulmonary oedema or potentially scarring from previous tissue damage, which when present can affect the lung's ability to expand, limiting the tidal volume and reducing the capability to deliver medications. Several structures act as natural immune defences and along with mucociliary clearance, drug deposition is likely to be further reduced.

---

### PAUSE AND REFLECT 2.5

Consider the different routes of drug administration that you have seen. Reflect on the advantages and disadvantages of oral, intravenous and topical routes. Can you think why these drugs were administered by this specific route?

---

## CHAPTER SUMMARY

Chapter 2 has focused on the first stage of pharmacokinetics – drug absorption. The different routes of drug administration employed in medicine management have been explained with respect to normal physiology. Whilst the aim of drug absorption is to ensure that the drug reaches the systemic circulation so it can be distributed around the body, there are many factors which impact the rate and extent of drug absorption. Whilst not exhaustive, these relate to the physiological barriers the drug needs to navigate, the formulation of the drug, the physical and chemical properties of the drug, the presence of disease and age-related changes.

# DRUG DISTRIBUTION 3

---
### LEARNING OUTCOMES
---

By the end of this chapter, you should be able to:

1 Explore the pharmacological concept of drug distribution
2 Critically examine the factors which affect the movement of drugs across body compartments
3 Discuss related concepts: plasma protein binding, bioavailability, drug distribution and the clinical implications relating to drug safety and therapeutics

---

## INTRODUCTION

This chapter aims to explore the second stage of the pharmacokinetic process – drug distribution.

## DEFINITION OF DRUG DISTRIBUTION

Drug distribution is the second stage of the pharmacokinetic process and refers to the circulation and deposition of the drug throughout the human body, once the drug has entered the circulatory system.

The molecular structure of drugs varies significantly, and their physical and chemical composition will influence the extent to which drug molecules are able to move from the circulatory system, across capillary and cellular membranes, or in the case of drugs which affect the central nervous system, navigate the blood–brain barrier.

Chemically, drugs may have polar properties in that they dissolve well in water, termed *hydrophilic*, or alternatively do not but are able to dissolve in lipids (i.e. are lipid soluble or lipophilic). It is common for drugs to have both hydrophilic and lipophilic properties. It is these properties which predict the extent to which a drug moves out of the blood and is able to navigate cell membranes (Table 3.1).

**Table 3.1** Properties of common drugs

| | |
|---|---|
| Hydrophilic (water soluble drugs) | B-Lactam antimicrobial: penicillin, amoxicillin |
| | Aminoglycosides – e.g. gentamicin |
| Lipophilic (lipid soluble drugs) | Macrolides – e.g. clarithromycin |
| | General anaesthetics |
| | Benzodiazepines – e.g. diazepam |

In practice drugs are on a continuum between highly hydrophilic and lipophilic, with very few being at the ends of the spectrum.

### Highly Polar, Low Lipophilicity

Starting at the highly polar end, some drugs are highly polar and have low lipophilicity. These drugs tend to dissolve well in water but poorly in lipids. They may require specific transport mechanisms to cross lipid-rich biological barriers like cell membranes. Examples include some antibiotics and certain neurotransmitters.

### Moderately Polar, Moderate Lipophilicity

Most drugs are moderately polar and have moderate lipophilicity. Most drugs fall into this category. This balance between polarity and lipophilicity, allows them to distribute throughout both aqueous and lipid environments to some extent. These drugs can often cross cell membranes and distribute evenly throughout the body. Many commonly prescribed medications, such as beta-blockers, **analgesics** and **antihistamines**, fit into this category.

### Low Polarity, High Lipophilicity

Then, at the other end of the continuum, we have low polarity drugs. Some drugs are highly lipophilic and have low polarity. These drugs tend to dissolve well in lipids but poorly in water. They can easily cross cell membranes and distribute into fatty tissues. Examples include some anaesthetics and many psychoactive drugs.

## THE VOLUME OF DISTRIBUTION

The **volume of distribution** (VoD) of a drug is a theoretical term and pharmacokinetic concept. Although measured in litres, it is important to note that the VoD is not an actual physiological volume, otherwise it can be confusing when VoDs more than the volume of fluid in the human body are presented.

Calculating the VoD can help understand the extent to which a drug is distributed within the body following entry into the systemic circulation. Physiological changes resulting from disease and age can affect the distribution of a drug.

A drug's VoD is thought of in relation to the following body compartments, introduced in Chapter 1:

- Extracellular fluid, which comprises the plasma (5 litres) and all other fluid compartments outside the cell (total approximately 10 litres)
- Intracellular fluid (approximately 30 litres)
- Muscle (equivalent to 100 litres)
- Adipose tissue (i.e. fat; equivalent to 1000 litres)

These values may differ slightly in publications but remember that it is the relative magnitude of the different numbers rather than the exact values.

To understand the concept of VoD it can help to start with a simple container model. This can help develop our understanding of how VoD is calculated. If we take the same concentration of a drug, 100 mg, and inject it into three different sized volumes of fluid, it makes sense that the drug will be most diluted in the largest volume. If we were then to take a sample from each of the containers, we could tell which one was from the smallest container (highest concentration, the least diluted) and which was from the largest (lowest concentration, the most diluted). You can imagine then that a drug that gets into all the compartments of the body would be the most diluted and a drug that remains in the blood would be the least diluted (see Figure 3.1).

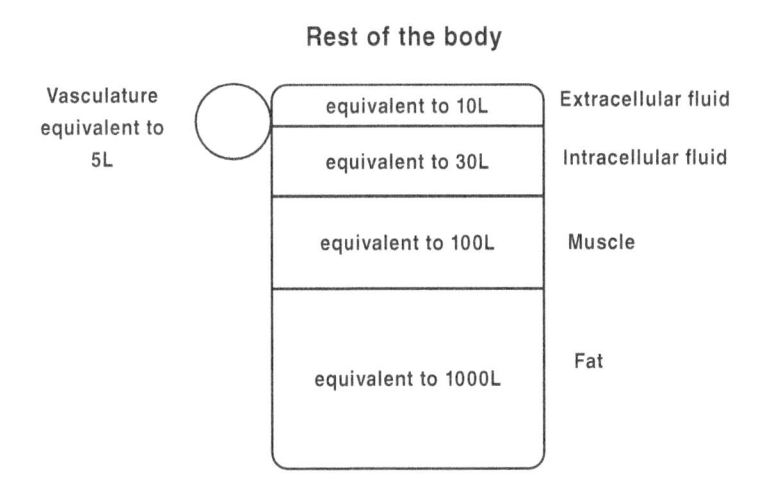

**Figure 3.1** A simple compartment model of VoD

This principle helps generate a formula and a method of working out the VoD. If a fixed bolus dose of a drug is injected and a blood sample is taken, a calculation can be made to establish how extensively or not the drug is distributed throughout the body compartments.

The dose of the drug will always be known as will the plasma concentration, but the 'size' of the container is not known. However, knowing the container's size will help understand the extent of the drug's distribution within the body.

The formula is:

> administered dose of the drug = volume of distribution × plasma concentration

The equation can be rearranged, so the volume of distribution is on the left:

$$\text{volume of distribution (VoD)} = \frac{\text{the administered dose of the drug}}{\text{plasma concentration}}$$

Now we know that the larger the number we get out of this equation, the larger the VoD and the more the drug is extensively distributed throughout the body compartments. Pharmacologists help our understanding by linking the VoD to which compartment the drug is primarily located. For example, if 100mg of a drug is injected into the bloodstream and a blood sample measures the drug concentration to be 20 mg/L, the volume of distribution (VoD) would be 5 litres:

$$\text{volume of distribution (VoD)} = \frac{\text{administered dose of the drug}}{\text{plasma concentration}}$$

$$\text{VoD} = \frac{100 \text{ mg}}{20 \text{ mg/L}} = 5 \text{ litres}$$

This tells us that because we have approximately 5 litres of blood plasma, it is almost exclusively contained in the circulatory system. In this case the numbers make sense and relate directly to the physiological volume.

Interestingly, if the value came out lower than this, it would probably mean that the drug is trapped somewhere in the blood that does not then get measured when a sample is taken. Very low VoDs can therefore be an indication of drugs that are highly protein bound. A very low VoD doesn't make sense physiologically because we still have the same 5 litres of blood, but remember VoD is a not a physiological volume, just the results of a calculation that can tell us something about the pharmacokinetic characteristics of a drug.

Let's look at the other end of the scale where there is a very large volume of distribution. In this case we will inject the same amount of drug (i.e. 100 mg) and measure the concentration in the plasma to be 0.1 mg/L.

$$\text{volume of distribution (VoD)} = \frac{\text{administered dose of the drug}}{\text{plasma concentration}}$$

$$\text{VoD} = \frac{100\,\text{mg}}{0.1\,\text{mg/L}} = 1{,}000 \text{ litres}$$

The VoD is 1,000 litres and of course we do not have this amount of fluid in the body. However, pharmacologically, a very large VoD means the drug has readily left the circulatory system and been extensively distributed to all parts of the body, particularly the fat compartment, so much so that it prefers this compartment to the blood compartment.

To note, the volume of distribution of a drug is calculated based on a man who weighs 70 kg.

*Drugs with a high volume of distribution include:*

Propranolol: 270 litres/70 kg

Digoxin: 500 litres/70 kg

Meperidine: 310 litres/70 kg

*Drugs with a low volume of distribution include:*

Aspirin: 11 litres/70 kg

Tolbutamide: 7 litres/70 kg

Warfarin: 9.8 litres/70 kg

Gentamicin: 20 litres/70 kg

So, what makes a drug go where? The overall driving factor in this case is the relative fat or water solubility of the drug. This is sometimes referred to as how polar (hydrophilic) the drug is or how non-polar (lipophilic) the drug is. Some highly water-soluble drugs such as the penicillin group stay mainly in the fluid compartments (blood, ECF and ICF) whereas highly lipid soluble drugs, which can move through cell membranes, such as general anaesthetics and benzodiazepines, distribute more widely and extensively into fat.

So, you can now see that the volume of distribution can give you an indication of where the drug is distributed within the body, how extensively and what chemical characteristics the drug might possess.

## PAUSE AND REFLECT 3.1

How does the concept of volume of distribution help us understand the distribution of a drug within the body and its relationship to plasma concentration?

### So, What Use Is VoD?

Understanding a drug's VoD can help us understand the impact of an individual's physiology on drug distribution through the body, the relative drug levels and consequently whether dose adjustments are necessary. The VoD can also help us understand what loading dose may need to be administered to achieve a therapeutic plasma concentration.

Let's say we want to get an initial target drug concentration of 5 mg/L in the plasma, and we know the VoD of the drug is 1,000 litres (this would be a drug distributing extensively and in fats). The loading dose is calculated to be 5 g (see the calculation below).

> loading dose (LD) = amount of drug in the body
> loading dose (LD) = VoD × plasma concentration
> LD = 1,000 litres x 5 mg/L
> **LD = 5,000 mg = 5 g**

Conversely if we take a hydrophilic drug (i.e. a drug which remains in the plasma of the blood and therefore has a much lower VoD of 5 litres) and want the same target drug concentration of 5 mg/L, the loading dose is much lower at 25 mg.

> loading dose (LD) = amount of drug in the body
> loading dose (LD) = VoD x plasma concentration
> LD = 5 litres x 5 mg/L
> **LD = 25 mg**

## FACTORS WHICH INFLUENCE THE VOLUME OF DISTRIBUTION OF A DRUG

There are several factors which influence the VoD of a drug. The molecular structure of a drug and its associated lipophilic and hydrophilic properties determine the extent to which a drug moves from the systemic circulation across cell membranes to effect therapeutic action.

As discussed in Chapter 1, a lipophilic (fat soluble) drug is a nonpolar compound which can diffuse readily across the fatty bilayer of the cell membranes, whereas polar drugs (i.e. hydrophilic drugs) are insoluble in water and therefore cross cell membranes via facilitated transport. As a result, they are not widely distributed in the body.

## Body-Related Factors and an Individual's Physiology

If a drug's VoD is known to be large, it can be assumed it will be extensively distributed to body fat. However, if this drug is administered to an individual who is clinically obese, a higher dose will be required in comparison to someone who is the same body weight but has a higher muscle mass ratio. This could be important, for example, when giving a general anaesthetic, a lipophilic drug which must traverse the central nervous system to affect consciousness. Unfortunately, a lipophilic drug will also be reservoired in other fatty stores (e.g. adipose tissue) throughout the body, which will mean the anaesthetic effect is prolonged, the person will take longer to regain consciousness and risk associated post-anaesthetic complications.

With advancing age, the composition of body water in comparison to body fat changes. In the older person, the relative proportion of body fat increases whilst there is a diminution of total body water (i.e. muscle mass). The changes in the proportion of body water versus body fat with advancing age can affect the distribution of drugs within these compartments. For example, for drugs which are highly hydrophilic (e.g. digoxin, prescribed for atrial fibrillation), the reduction of total body water seen in the older person can affect the concentration of the drug. If we effectively reduce the total volume of distribution of body water, then digoxin will be more concentrated in the plasma and risk toxicity.

Similarly, in physiological states and disease where there is a reduction of body water seen in dehydration and burns, for drugs which are hydrophilic the same scenario will occur. Conversely, in conditions where total body water is increased (e.g. oedema, ascites), hydrophilic drugs will be dispersed in a greater volume of water and therefore the plasma concentration will be lowered, potentially leading to therapeutic failure of the drug.

The relative decrease or increase in body fat will also be pharmacologically significant for drugs which are lipophilic.

As discussed, the dose of anaesthetic drugs must be adjusted to body weight. Because anaesthetic drugs must cross the blood–brain barrier and enter the fatty substance of the brain, they also 'sequent' into other fatty areas of the body (e.g. adipose tissue). There is a risk that lipid-soluble drugs may accumulate, and the half-life be extended, which risks toxicity. Elderly people are particularly susceptible to the sedating effects of benzodiazepines for this reason.

During pregnancy, blood volume can increase by 40%, peaking at 28–34 weeks' gestation, and total body water by 6–8 litres, both altering plasma drug levels.

In disease there may be a loss of the integrity of the cell membrane so that the fluid compartments are compromised. In severe burns, for example, drugs will leak out in serous fluid. Other structures limit the extent of drug distribution. A good example is the blood–brain barrier (BBB).

## The Blood-Brain Barrier

The brain holds a unique status as a protected site within the body, prioritised above other organs. This safeguarding is achieved through the evolution of the blood-brain barrier (BBB). The BBB is a specialised structure consisting of fully differentiated brain endothelial cells in the neurovascular system (see Figure 3.2). Its primary role is to separate circulating blood components from neurons, thereby preserving the chemical composition of the neuronal microenvironment. This stable microenvironment is crucial for the optimal functioning of neuronal circuits, synaptic transmission, synaptic remodelling, angiogenesis and neurogenesis. Additionally, the BBB acts as a defence mechanism, shielding the brain from pathogens and providing it with a relative immune privilege.

The BBB comprises densely packed brain endothelial cells interconnected by tight junctions, inhibiting the passage of molecules and ions in an effective way. Furthermore, this barrier is regulated by efflux transporters, acting as vigilant gatekeepers. An example of such a transporter is the transmembrane protein P-glycoprotein (P-gp), ubiquitously present in the membranes of the intestine, liver, kidney and the blood–brain barrier.

These proteins serve a crucial role by expelling foreign molecules that approach the barrier, a protective mechanism designed to prevent the ingress of toxins and undesired substances into the brain. However, this defensive function may inadvertently extend to the removal of drug molecules, potentially hindering therapeutic efficacy. Notably, the recently discovered efflux pump BCRP (breast cancer resistance protein) has been identified within the blood–brain barrier. Originally detected in breast cancer cells, BCRP is implicated in conferring resistance to anti-cancer drugs.

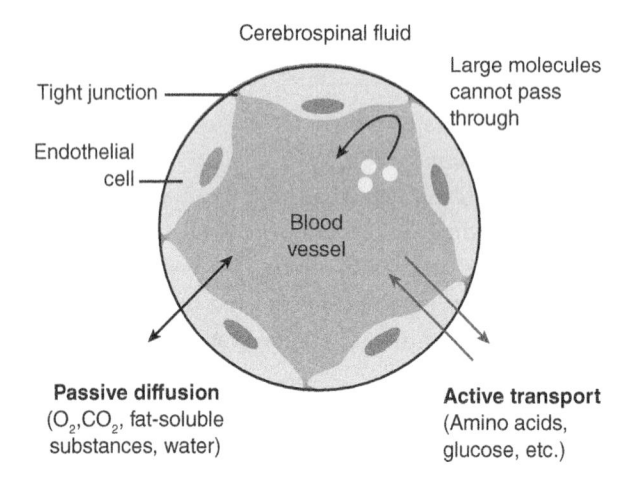

**Figure 3.2** Brain and behaviour

The BBB is a major obstacle for drug delivery to the brain and 98% of small molecule drugs that currently exist are excluded as are almost all the larger more water-soluble ones. By studying the BBB scientists can look for ways to deliver drugs to the brain and bypass the barrier. Equally important is the study of the pathophysiology of the BBB because when this changes, drugs that do not normally reach the brain will do, and whilst this may be advantageous it may also be problematic. For example, in the case of meningitis, an initial treatment may be a single dose of 1,200mg of benzylpenicillin. This is a relatively large water-soluble molecule which would not normally penetrate the BBB. However, in meningitis, the meninges and the BBB become more permeable due to inflammation and the antibiotic can reach its target site of action. Conversely, several of the antihistamine **antagonist** drugs must be used cautiously in older people. Whilst they are relatively water insoluble drugs and do not penetrate the BBB, decreased cholinergic neurons or receptors in the brain, reduced hepatic and renal function and increased blood–brain permeability make older people sensitive to the central nervous system and anticholinergic-related side effects (e.g. sedation).

### Physiological Changes that Can Modulate the Blood-Brain Barrier

Some diseases or physiological situations can change the permeability of the BBB. This is either by making it more permeable or making the transporters in the BBB that move molecules in and out act differently, either up-regulating them so they work more effectively or down-regulating them, doing the opposite. If inflammation of the brain occurs, the blood–brain barrier's tight junctions may open, playing a role in the development of brain oedema. Similarly, during physiological stressors such as starvation or hypoxia, GLUT1 transporters, which transport glucose into the brain, are upregulated to meet increased energy demands. As a final example, certain inflammatory mediators (e.g. histamine and bradykinin) heighten capillary permeability on the endothelium of the brain, just as they do in other parts of the body.

These changes can result in drugs that might not usually get into the brain, making drug effects unpredictable. In fact, a whole host of diseases can change the permeability of the blood–brain barrier such as stroke, trauma, infections, tumours, multiple sclerosis, HIV, Alzheimer's disease, Parkinson's disease, epilepsy and even inflammatory-related pain.

Because the effects of chronic conditions on the BBB have not been extensively studied, the effects of changes in the BBB are difficult to predict. However, we do understand the basic characteristics of drugs which can navigate the BBB successfully. Drugs designed to treat mental illnesses like schizophrenia and depression consist of small-molecule, lipid-soluble compounds, or individual ions which enable them to traverse the BBB effectively and reach their target sites within the brain. On the other hand, some other drugs that treat central nervous system (CNS) diseases don't have these characteristics – for example, large enzymes that might treat Alzheimer's disease, Huntington's disease, and Parkinson's disease. In the case of Parkinson's disease, levodopa or variations used to alleviate symptoms are small molecule and lipid-soluble molecules and can enter the brain but sadly provide only temporary relief.

### Loperamide: An Example

Loperamide is used to treat diarrhoea and is an opioid drug. At low doses, loperamide acts locally on the gastrointestinal tract. Loperamide is a lipophilic molecule, but it has a structure which reduces its lipid solubility and increases its molecular size compared to other opioids. Unlike other opioids, this limits its ability to cross the BBB, and so even at high doses, side effects of respiratory depression or euphoria are unlikely. Importantly, any loperamide that does enter the barrier is pumped back out. Loperamide is a substrate for P-glycoprotein, an efflux pump located on the luminal surface of brain capillary endothelial cells forming the BBB. P-glycoprotein actively transports substrates, including loperamide, back into the bloodstream, reducing the drug's concentration in the brain.

> **PAUSE AND REFLECT 3.2**
>
> Consider the factors that can affect the volume of distribution of a drug. How do these factors impact upon drug levels and drug efficacy?

## PLASMA PROTEIN BINDING

Plasma protein binding refers to the degree to which a drug is attached or bound to plasma proteins found in the blood.

Blood is made up of several components, with the largest being the plasma. Plasma is composed of approximately 93% water and electrolytes with plasma proteins making up a further 7%. Plasma proteins are responsible for controlling oncotic pressure, transporting substances, coagulation and promoting inflammation.

Plasma proteins also bind to many drugs, with drugs present within blood being in either a bound or unbound state.

The most significant plasma proteins involved in drug binding are albumin, alpha 1-acid glycoprotein, and lipoproteins. Albumin is the most abundant plasma protein, and it binds mainly to acidic drugs, e.g. non-steroidal anti-inflammatory drugs such as Ibuprofen, whilst alpha 1-acid glycoproteins, lipoproteins or both bind to basic drugs.

Once a drug binds to a protein it forms a protein–drug complex. This protein–drug complex is then too large to pass through cell membranes, therefore only a free or 'unbound' drug is available for delivery to the tissues to produce the necessary pharmacological effect (see Figure 3.3). The degree of protein binding can greatly affect the pharmacokinetics of drugs (not only distribution but metabolism and excretion too) and therefore drug efficacy.

Plasma protein binding is reversible in most cases; therefore, a chemical equilibrium will exist between the bound and unbound states:

DRUG (unbound, active) + PROTEIN ↔ DRUG–PROTEIN COMPLEX
(inactive drug)

It is the unbound fraction or free drug that exhibits pharmacological effects and provides the therapeutic action of the drug. It is also the fraction that will be metabolised and/or excreted. For example, the 'fraction bond' of the anticoagulant warfarin is 97%.

This means that of the total amount of warfarin in the blood, 97% of it is bound to plasma proteins. The other 3% (the unbound fraction) is the amount that is active, and it will exhibit its pharmacological effect. This is also the amount of drug available for metabolism and excretion. Conversely, the less bound a drug is, the more readily it will cross a cell membrane. For lithium, a drug used to stabilise mood disorders, the unbound fraction is 100% and does not bind to plasma proteins at all. Therefore, all of the drug will be available to exert its pharmacological effect and the dose will not be affected by variation in an individual's plasma protein levels.

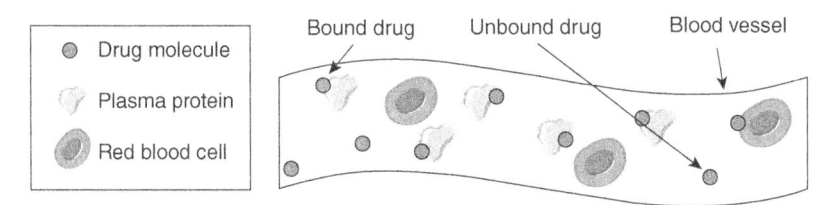

**Figure 3.3** Drug distribution

Source: Created using Servier Medical Art. Servier Medical Art is licenced under a Creative Commons Attribution 3.0 Unported License https://creativecommons.org/licenses/by/3.0/.

The extent of drug distribution is affected by plasma protein binding. Drugs that are highly protein-bound have a lower distribution volume because they remain in the bloodstream. For example, warfarin, an anticoagulant medication, is highly protein-bound (approximately 97%) to albumin in the bloodstream. Therefore, changes in plasma protein levels or binding **affinity** can affect the distribution of warfarin and its pharmacological effects. Drugs that are less bound to proteins have a higher distribution volume and are therefore more readily available for tissue uptake.

Changes in plasma protein levels or binding affinity can alter drug distribution, leading to potential changes in drug efficacy and toxicity.

Protein binding can also influence the drug's biological half-life. The bound drug–protein complex may act as a reservoir or depot from which the drug can be slowly released. Since the unbound form is being metabolised and/or excreted from the body, the bound fraction will be released to maintain equilibrium. This can be clinically significant for antimicrobial therapy. Some antimicrobials utilise a high degree of protein binding which serve as a drug depot, prolonging the time that the antimicrobial remains above the necessary concentration to inhibit bacterial growth. This improves the efficacy of the drug.

## Factors That Affect Plasma Protein Binding

There are several factors that may impact plasma protein binding and result in a biological effect for the individual. These include factors that affect the concentrations of free drug, the number of plasma proteins available and their affinity for the drug.

## Saturation of the Plasma Protein Binding Sites

The amount of bound drug in high drug concentrations can reach an upper limit, determined by the number of available binding sites. As the concentration of a drug in plasma increases, binding sites on proteins are increasingly saturated and this can result in unwanted higher percentages of unbound drug in the plasma. Examples of the drugs that do this are ceftriaxone and cefazolin, both of which are cephalosporin antibiotics used to treat bacterial infection.

## Competition for Binding Sites

A drug will sometimes compete for plasma proteins binding sites with other drugs or endogenous compounds. Let's take two drugs: drug A and drug B. If drug A has a greater affinity for plasma proteins than drug B, then it will compete for the binding sites. As a result, drug B will be displaced from the plasma protein binding sites. Free, unbound levels of drug B will rise, which risks drug toxicity and possibly adverse drug reactions. It would be even more concerning if drug B had a narrow **therapeutic index**. Narrow therapeutic index drugs (NTIDs) have a narrow range between the effective therapeutic dose and the toxic dose. Examples of these drugs are digoxin (a drug used to improve the efficiency of the heart) and warfarin (a drug used for its anticoagulant effect). A sudden increase in the unbound fraction of these drugs may provide a toxic effect. This can lead to clinical consequences such as risk of bleeding tendencies with warfarin and severe cardiac arrythmia with digoxin.

Such changes in protein binding caused by drug interactions are assumed to instantaneously change free drug concentrations and have been frequently documented as the cause of adverse drug reactions. However, often the increase in free drug concentration is fleeting, as drug distribution and drug elimination will compensate to maintain therapeutic plasma concentrations of the drug.

Drugs may also compete with endogenous substances. For example, when sulfonamide competitively binds to plasma proteins, it reduces albumin's affinity for bilirubin, releasing free bilirubin and increasing the risk of bilirubin encephalopathy in newborn babies.

## Age

There are plasma protein changes along the age spectrum. In elderly people, albumin levels are decreased but alpha 1-acid glycoprotein levels are generally not altered. However, changes in protein binding in old age are not usually clinically important in drug therapy. Rather, it is physiological and pathophysiological changes that may occur more often in elderly people that produce more clinically significant changes. These changes may include compromised liver and renal function and decreased cardiac output. Therefore, it is important to understand the relationship between the physiology of ageing, disease and protein binding to provide effective drug therapy. Monitoring of unbound drug concentrations helps to provide fundamental information needed for the dosage regimen. However, the pharmacological therapy for elderly people should be individualised considering all these factors.

In neonates, plasma protein levels are lower and gradually increase with age, reaching adult levels at about 10–12 months. At birth, albumin concentrations are 75–80% of adult levels whilst alpha 1-acid glycoprotein is initially half adult levels, which could lead to an increased fraction of unbound drug for some drugs, particularly those that bind to alpha 1-acid glycoproteins. Moreover, drugs that bind to plasma proteins seem to be more vulnerable to displacement by endogenous compounds such as bilirubin and fatty acids, which are found in high concentrations in newborn babies. Displacement of the medication can cause an increase in free drug concentration, which may produce undesirable effects. Alternatively, sulfonamide competes to bind to plasma proteins and reduces albumin's affinity for bilirubin. This increases the amount of free bilirubin, increasing the risk of bilirubin encephalopathy in neonates.

## Ethnicity

Ethnic differences have been found for plasma protein-binding in the two major drug-binding proteins, alpha 1-acid glycoprotein (AGP) and albumin. Studies show that ethnic differences for drugs which bind exclusively to albumin (e.g. acids) are rare. However ethnic differences in plasma protein-binding of drugs to AGP appear to be quite common. It has been found that the plasma concentration of alpha 1-acid glycoproteins is significantly lower in people of Asian rather than European or African descent. East Asian patients may require lower dosages of psychotropic drugs, such as antipsychotics, lithium and antidepressants, than non-Asian patients (Lin, 2022). This can be partly explained by low levels of alpha-acid glycoproteins, which provide binding sites for psychotropic drugs. If there are fewer plasma protein binding sites, less of the drug will be bound, and more will be free and therefore active. Thus, the dosage may require adjusting to a lesser amount.

## Disease

Plasma protein levels may decrease due to malnutrition or hepatic disease, as plasma proteins are produced in the liver. Additionally, renal diseases such as glomerulonephritis or nephrotic syndrome can result in the loss of albumin, further reducing plasma protein levels.

In all these instances, the outcome is a smaller proportion of drug in bound form and more free drug in the plasma. The greater amount of free drug can produce a greater therapeutic effect and reduced drug dosages may therefore be indicated. However, in clinical practice the implications of the reduction of plasma proteins on drug efficacy, risk of toxicity or potential interactions with other drugs is not fully understood and needs further exploration.

For instance, hypoalbuminemia, which occurs in conditions like liver disease or malnutrition, can lead to increased levels of free (unbound) warfarin, potentially increasing the risk of bleeding due to its anticoagulant effects.

# FACTORS WHICH AFFECT DRUG DISTRIBUTION

There are a number of factors that affect drug distribution, which we will now explore.

## Drug-Related Factors

Drug-related factors that affect drug distribution include:

- pH
- Perfusion
- Molecular size

### pH

The pH of tissues and body fluids can affect drug distribution by influencing the degree of ionisation of the drug molecule. Drugs that are weak acids or bases tend to ionise in response to changes in pH, which can affect their ability to cross cell membranes and penetrate tissues. For example, acidic drugs are more likely to be ionised in alkaline environments and vice versa, impacting their distribution into tissues with different pH levels. For example, morphine is a weak base that can exist in both ionised and non-ionised forms depending on the pH of its environment. In acidic environments, such as the stomach, morphine tends to be non-ionised and more readily absorbed. However, in alkaline environments, such as the small intestine, morphine becomes ionised and less likely to cross cell membranes. In practice this is likely to be important only if the patient already has specific gastrointestinal pathophysiology. Variations in pH along the gastrointestinal tract can affect the absorption and distribution of morphine, influencing its pharmacological effects.

### Perfusion

Perfusion refers to blood flow to tissues, which plays a crucial role in drug distribution. Highly perfused tissues, such as the liver, kidneys and brain, receive a greater supply of blood and therefore have higher rates of drug delivery compared to less perfused tissues. Variations in tissue perfusion can affect the distribution of drugs to different organs and tissues, influencing their pharmacological effects. Propofol, an anaesthetic, is highly perfused in tissues with high blood flow, such as the heart and brain. Its rapid distribution to these tissues allows for effective and rapid anaesthesia during procedures. However, propofol's distribution into and out of poorly perfused tissues, such as fat, is slower, leading to prolonged systemic effects and potential toxicity if not adequately monitored.

A reduction in arterial blood flow – seen, for example, in vascular disorders – will inevitably reduce drug delivery. As an example, intravenous antimicrobial drugs will not be delivered to an infected necrotic toe; hence the need for topical applications.

## Molecular Size

The molecular size of a drug molecule can influence its distribution within the body. Small molecules can penetrate cell membranes more easily and distribute more readily into tissues compared to larger molecules. Drugs with larger molecular sizes may be restricted to certain compartments or tissues with larger interstitial spaces, affecting their distribution kinetics and tissue penetration.

## Body-Related Factors

Body-related factors include:

- Fat/water ratio
- Age-related changes
- Disease

### Fat/Water Ratio

The distribution of drugs within the body is influenced by the relative proportions of fat and water in different tissues. Lipophilic drugs tend to distribute more readily into fatty tissues, while hydrophilic drugs have greater distribution into water-rich tissues. Variations in body composition, such as changes in fat mass or hydration status, can impact the distribution of drugs and their concentration profiles in different tissues. For example, propofol has a high lipid solubility and tends to distribute across lipid-based barriers such as the blood–brain barrier. This distribution pattern contributes to propofol's rapid onset of action and short duration of effect, as it is quickly redistributed from the central nervous system to peripheral tissues. Therefore, variations in body fat content can impact the distribution kinetics of propofol, affecting its pharmacological profile and dosing requirements.

### Age-Related Changes

Age-related changes in body composition, organ function and blood flow can affect drug distribution patterns. For example, changes in fat mass and lean body mass with age can alter the volume of distribution of lipophilic and hydrophilic drugs. Additionally, age-related changes in organ function, such as decreased renal and hepatic clearance, can affect drug distribution and elimination kinetics. For example, digoxin, a medication used to treat heart failure and atrial fibrillation, has a narrow therapeutic index and is primarily eliminated by renal excretion. Decreased glomerular filtration rate and renal blood flow can lead to reduced clearance of digoxin in older adults. As a result, older patients may be at higher risk of digoxin toxicity due to prolonged drug accumulation and reduced ability to eliminate the drug from the body.

### Disease

Certain diseases and conditions can alter body water distribution and affect drug distribution patterns. For instance, conditions that result in loss of body water, such as dehydration, burns or third-spacing (accumulation of fluid in interstitial spaces), can lead to changes in drug concentration gradients and distribution volumes. Similarly, diseases affecting organ function, such as renal or hepatic impairment, can impact drug distribution kinetics and tissue penetration. Vancomycin, an antibiotic used to treat serious bacterial infections, exhibits altered distribution in patients with renal impairment. Reduced renal function can lead to decreased clearance of vancomycin, resulting in higher plasma concentrations and potentially increased distribution to tissues. In patients with renal dysfunction, dose adjustments are necessary to prevent drug accumulation and toxicity.

## CHAPTER SUMMARY

Chapter 3 has addressed the second stage of pharmacokinetics: drug distribution. The pharmacokinetics value 'volume of distribution' is explained relative to the fluid compartments in the body and the physiological barriers that influence the movement of drugs across these barriers. The influence of disease, body-related differences, and a drug's physical and chemical properties are explained. Plasma protein binding, a pharmacological principle which affects the 'free drug' dosage that is circulated, is explained, as are the factors which may affect drug availability.

# DRUG METABOLISM 4

---
### LEARNING OUTCOMES
---

By the end of this chapter, you should be able to:

1. Explore the pharmacological concept and principles of drug metabolism (biotransformation)
2. Discuss the sites of drug metabolism and the physiological mechanisms involved in the metabolic processes
3. Critically examine the drug-related and physiological factors which affect the rate and extent of drug metabolism
4. Discuss the clinical applications of drug metabolism with respect to a drug's safety profile and preparation for excretion
5. Explain the pharmacokinetics principles: half-life, steady state levels, therapeutic index in the context of safe and therapeutic drug levels

---

## INTRODUCTION

This chapter aims to explore the third stage of the pharmacokinetic process – drug metabolism.

## CONCEPTS AND PRINCIPLES OF DRUG METABOLISM

The processes involved in drug metabolism prepare the drug for excretion, which is important in ensuring that drug levels remain safe and therapeutic. Drug metabolism principally occurs in the liver but there are other sites of drug metabolism or **biotransformation**, which include, for example, the intestinal wall, blood plasma, lungs and kidneys.

There are drugs, however, that are excreted by the body unchanged and therefore do not undergo metabolism (e.g. gentamicin, digoxin).

There are principally two phases of drug metabolism:

- First-pass metabolism
- Final metabolism

## First-Pass Metabolism

As explained in Chapter 3, all orally administered drugs which enter the mesenteric blood vessels from the ileum (small intestine) drain into the hepatic portal vein. In its role as a detoxifying organ, the liver will, to a greater or lesser extent, metabolise the drug as it first 'passes through'. For some drugs (e.g. morphine sulphate) the extent of first-pass metabolism is significant in that only approximately 24% of the administered dose leaves the liver via the hepatic vein to enter the systemic circulation. This means that for drugs with a high rate of first-pass metabolism, the oral dose is much larger than the intravenous dose to achieve therapeutic levels.

## Final Drug Metabolism

Drug metabolism is the third stage of the pharmacokinetic process, but it is important to acknowledge that because blood flows through the liver during every cardiac cycle, the metabolism of a drug is a continuous process, such that the action of the drug is taking place simultaneously.

### Anatomy and Physiology of the Liver

The liver is in the upper right-hand quadrant of the abdomen, beneath the diaphragm, and on top of the stomach, right kidney and intestines. It consists of two main lobes: the right and left lobe. There are two accessory lobes that arise from the larger right lobe known as the caudate and quadrate lobes (see Figure 4.1).

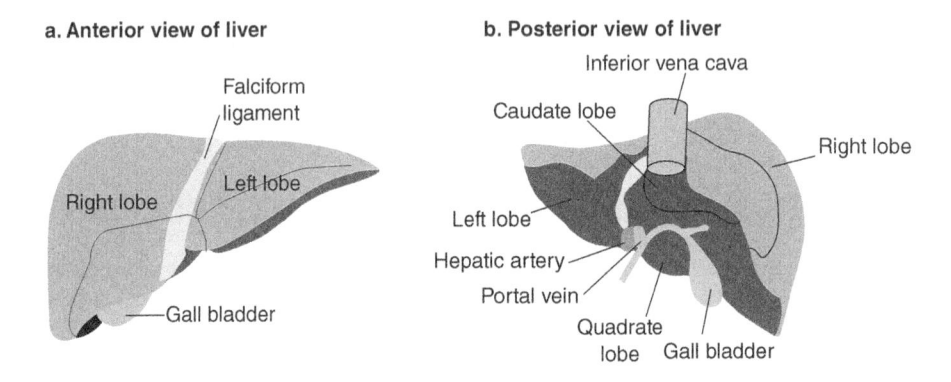

**Figure 4.1** Anatomy and physiology of the liver

It is a multi-faceted organ that carries out over 500 functions within the body, a number of which are explained below.

*Bile production and excretion*: The liver secretes 800 to 1,000 ml of bile into the small intestines. Bile contains bile salts needed for the digestion of dietary fats.

*Metabolism of fats, protein and carbohydrates*: Nutrients that enter the liver are broken down (metabolised) into products that are usable by the body cells, or they can be stored for future use.

*Storage of glycogen, vitamins and minerals*: Excess glucose is converted into glycogen and remains stored in the liver until it is required for energy production. Glycogen can be reconverted into glucose and released into the bloodstream to balance the blood glucose levels.

*Manufacture of blood serum proteins*: These include, for example, albumin and clotting proteins.

*Storage of iron*: The liver processes haemoglobin for use of its iron content.

*Clearance of bilirubin*: Bilirubin is a waste product produced by the breakdown of red blood cells. It is secreted by the liver into the gall bladder and mixed with bile, which empties into the intestines. Bilirubin is a yellowish, brown pigment and gives the faeces its colour. If there is a blockage in the gastrointestinal system, bilirubin accumulates and is absorbed into the bloodstream, resulting in a yellow tinge to the skin and conjunctiva of the eyes.

*Metabolism and detoxification*: The liver metabolises nitrogenous waste products and detoxifies harmful substances, including drugs.

The liver receives blood from two sources: the hepatic artery (which delivers oxygenated blood from the aorta) and the hepatic portal vein (delivering deoxygenated blood from the intestines that is high in nutrients). The hepatic portal system has two capillary beds. The first bed drains blood from the gastrointestinal tract and the other delivers the blood received in the hepatic sinusoids from the hepatic artery (see Figure 4.2).

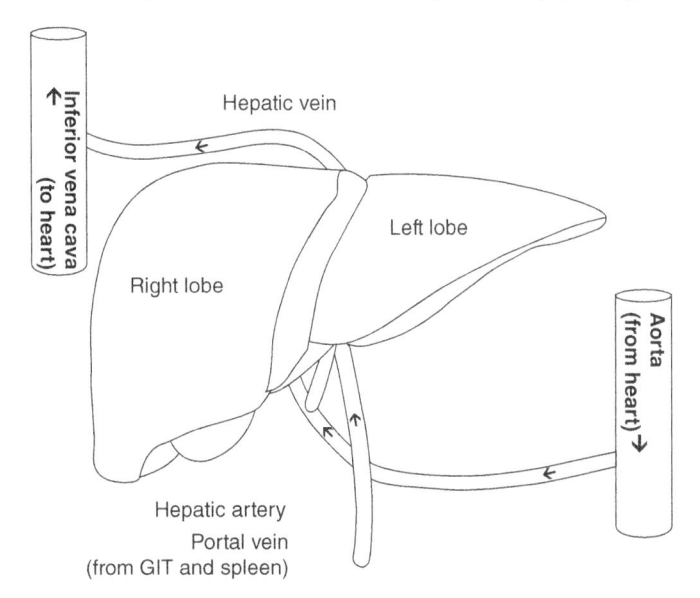

**Figure 4.2** How the liver receives blood

Nutrients and substances in the blood delivered to the liver via the hepatic portal vein are processed before they enter the systemic circulation. This action is very significant for drugs taken orally and leads to 'first-pass metabolism', a concept introduced in Chapter 2.

## THE ROLE OF THE CYTOCHROME P450 ENZYME SYSTEM

### Hepatic Enzymes

An important and vital function of the liver is the metabolism and/or detoxification of xenobiotics, the term given to foreign substances not normally found in the body, which includes drugs. The liver is the primary site for metabolism of drugs; however, enzymes involved in metabolism can also be found elsewhere, including the skin, lungs, gastrointestinal tract and kidneys (see Chapter 1 for a reminder of the action and role of enzymes).

Most drugs are lipophilic, which allows the drug to easily pass through cell membranes and have a therapeutic effect. However, lipophilic drugs are not easy to excrete. This is because lipophilic drugs will be reabsorbed from the nephron into the surrounding capillaries and re-enter the systemic circulation. They will therefore not be eliminated from the body.

'Metabolism' or 'biotransformation' are the terms used to describe the breakdown of drugs, which involves processes to convert drugs which are lipophilic into a more hydrophilic form. This will make them more susceptible to renal excretion as they will remain in the nephron tubule and be removed in the urine.

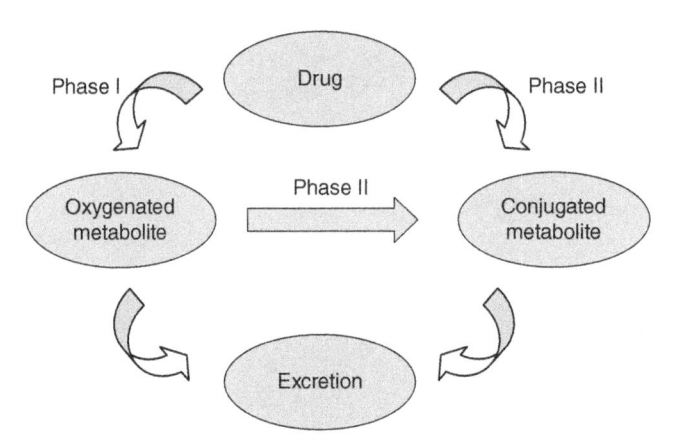

**Figure 4.3** The phases of drug metabolism

Drug metabolism has two mechanisms or processes: phase I and phase II. This suggests that drugs go through phase I first followed by phase II. However, several drugs may not undergo both processes to be metabolised (see Figure 4.3).

*Phase I metabolism* involves reactions that are catalysed by enzymes that bind oxygen, hydrogen, water or amino acids to the lipophilic drug molecule. These reactions either expose or introduce a polar functional group which increases the drug's water solubility (i.e. its hydrophilic properties).

These reactions include **hydrolysis**, reduction and **oxidation**.

- *Hydrolysis*: In a reaction with water, a bond in the drug is broken, resulting in two separate compounds. The water molecule also splits in two, with a hydrogen transferring to one of the compounds and a hydroxide to the other
- *Reduction*: Reactions resulting in the addition of hydrogen and/or the removal of oxygen
- *Oxidation*: Reactions resulting in the addition of oxygen and/or the removal of hydrogen

Oxidation reactions typically involve enzymes that belong to the cytochrome P450 class. Cytochrome P450 enzymes (sometimes abbreviated to CYP450) are a *microsomal super family of enzymes responsible for the biotransformation/metabolism of 75 % of all drugs. They are mostly abundant in the liver with different enzymes metabolising different drugs.*

Each enzyme is designated with the root symbol CYP for the superfamily, followed by a number indicating the gene family and a capital letter indicating the subfamily. Finally, a number for the specific gene is included. For example, the enzyme CYP2E1 is involved in paracetamol and alcohol metabolism, whilst CYP1A2 is involved in the metabolism of caffeine. CYP3A4 and CYP2D6 are the most significant enzymes, particularly CYP3A4 enzymes which are the most abundant in the CYP450 family.

Some products of oxidation and reduction reactions, however, require further modifications before they can be excreted and may undergo phase II metabolism.

In *phase II metabolism* conjugation reactions provide a further mechanism for preparing drugs for excretion. Substrates (substances on which an enzyme acts) for these reactions include both metabolites of the phase I reactions and compounds that already contain chemical groups appropriate for conjugation.

Conjugation reactions change compounds through attachment of hydrophilic groups, such as glucuronate, sulfate, glutathione and acetate to create more polar conjugates. This makes the **metabolite** ready for secretion into the blood or bile to be transported for excretion.

It is important to note that there are discussions within the world of pharmacology that hydrolysis is more closely related to conjugation than to oxidation or reduction and therefore should not be placed in phase I but rather be grouped with conjugation in phase II. However, for the purposes of this book we will use more traditional classifications as you will see these referred to in most of the pharmacological literature.

Most drugs, once they have undergone biotransformation produce inactive metabolites. However, some drugs, known as **pro-drugs**, are pharmacologically inactive until they are metabolised, and it is these metabolites that are active and produce the therapeutic effect. This will be explored in more detail later in this chapter.

An example of a pro-drug is codeine. Codeine has little or no analgesic activity until it is metabolised into morphine. It is metabolised by both phase I and phase II reactions. Approximately 80% of codeine is conjugated to form codeine-6-glucuronide, which may have some analgesic effects (phase I). However, typically less than 10% of codeine undergoes CYP2D6-mediated O-demethylation to the strong analgesic morphine (phase II).

## FACTORS THAT AFFECT DRUG METABOLISM

There are multiple factors that affect drug metabolism. These include genetics, age, sex, ethnicity and environmental factors as well as disease factors, inflammation, pregnancy, kidney and/or disease and drug–drug interactions.

### Genetics

Genetic factors may account for up to 95% of the variability of an individual's response to a drug. The study of genetic differences in response to drugs is called **pharmacogenetics**. Genes play a role in the production of enzymes, including those involved in drug metabolism. Genetic differences in these enzymes contribute to the variability in how individuals respond to and react to different drugs. Such differences can influence the amount of enzyme produced, as well as its function and activity rate.

As stated, genetic differences may change the number of enzymes that are available to metabolise drugs. For example, about 1 in 1,500 people have low levels of pseudocholinesterase. This is an enzyme that is primarily produced in the liver and is involved in a hydrolysis reaction that metabolises drugs such as succinylcholine and mivacurium. These are drugs sometimes given to temporarily relax muscles during surgery. If succinylcholine is not quickly metabolised, muscle relaxation may be prolonged for an individual and they may not be able to breathe on their own as normally expected following surgery. Therefore, the individual may require intubation and ventilation for a longer period.

Genetic differences in individuals may lead to metabolism of drugs at different rates. Some metabolise drugs very quickly. This rapid metabolism of a drug may result in the need for more frequent dosing or an increase in the dose to achieve the therapeutic effect. Some individuals may metabolise a drug so quickly that it is not therapeutic. Alternatively, if an individual metabolises a drug too slowly, the drug will accumulate in the body at normal dosages. A reduction in the dose or less frequent dosing will be required to avoid toxicity. This may be particularly concerning for drugs with a narrow margin of safety, such as phenytoin, prescribed for epilepsy. Phenytoin toxicity can result in adverse effects including ataxia, slurred speech, vomiting, lethargy, coma and even death.

Four types of phenotypical changes in CYP metabolism have been identified and defined in Table 4.1.

Table 4.1 Phenotypical changes in CYP metabolism

| Change | Effect on individual |
| --- | --- |
| Poor metabolisers (PM) | Usually experiences more adverse reactions at a normal dose of drug as medication is metabolised too slowly, resulting in toxicity |
| Intermediate metabolisers (IM) | Slow rate of drug metabolism may result in increased drug levels and occurrence of side effects |
| Extensive metabolisers (EM) | Normal rate of drug metabolism with expected drug levels |
| Ultra-rapid metabolisers (UM) | Drugs are rapidly metabolised resulting in sub-therapeutic drug levels and limited drug response |

The metaboliser types in Table 4.1 will influence how an individual will respond to a drug. Studies have shown that CYP2D6-poor metabolisers have poor analgesic response because of the reduced conversion of codeine to morphine. Conversely, CYP2D6-ultrarapid metabolisers quickly convert codeine to morphine and can experience an enhanced analgesic response (Dean and Kane, 2025).

A further example relates to the CYP2C19 gene which is known to encode a drug-metabolising enzyme that metabolises the **SSRIs** (selective serotonin re-uptake inhibitors) sertraline, citalopram and escitalopram amongst others, prescribed to manage anxiety and low mood. Poor metabolisers are at increased risk of adverse side effects due to a higher serum concentration of **antidepressant**. However, for ultrarapid metabolisers, the therapy is likely to be ineffective due to a decreased exposure to the drug. The recommendation for these patients would be to consider an alternative SSRI not metabolised by CYP2C19.

Figure 4.4 illustrates the different metaboliser types and their expected plasma concentration-time curves.

Pharmacogenetic testing may enable health professionals to understand why patients respond differently to certain drugs. This could aid decisions about therapy and lead to individualised therapeutic regimes. For example, patients who require azathioprine therapy are now routinely tested for thiopurine methyltransferase (TPMT) genotype to determine the most appropriate starting dose for drug therapy. Azathioprine is an immunosuppressant that helps control the immune system in inflammatory conditions such as rheumatoid arthritis, Crohn's disease and ulcerative colitis. Unfortunately, most genetic differences cannot be predicted before drug therapy, but for an increasing number of drugs (e.g. carbamazepine, clopidogrel and warfarin) changes in effectiveness and risk of toxicity have been specifically associated with certain genetic variations.

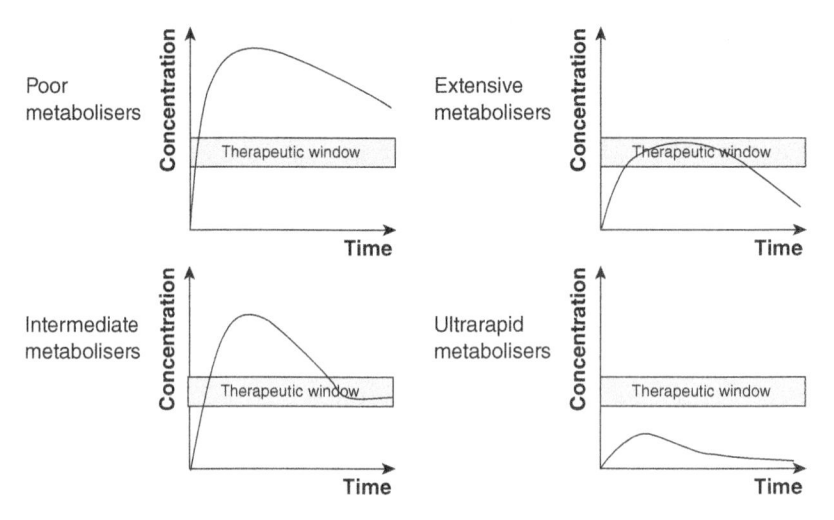

**Figure 4.4** Different metaboliser types and their expected plasma concentration-time curves

---

### PAUSE AND REFLECT 4.1

How do genetic differences in CYP450 affect drug metabolism, drug levels and therefore patient outcomes?

---

## Age

The age of an individual can influence hepatic enzyme function and therefore the rate and extent of drug metabolism.

With advancing age, the liver's capacity for metabolism through the CYP450 system reduces. This is due to decreased hepatic volume and blood flow. Therefore, drugs are metabolised at a slower rate and may lead to the drug remaining in the circulation for longer than expected, prolonging the half-life and resulting in toxicity.

However, ageing does not impact drugs that are metabolised by conjugation only.

At the other end of the age spectrum, neonates and babies under six months have an underdeveloped hepatic enzyme system due to liver volume and along with reduced hepatic blood flow, hepatic metabolism will be reduced. As a result, there will need to be dose reduction and caution with drug dosing. This can be illustrated by the administration of chloramphenicol, an antibiotic. Chloramphenicol is metabolised by a conjugation reaction, but this pathway is slow in neonates. Therefore, the drug may remain in the circulation in higher than expected concentrations. Excessively high serum levels of chloramphenicol have been linked to 'grey baby syndrome' which results in circulatory collapse that can have fatal consequences.

## Sex

The sex of an individual may affect drug metabolism. Oestrogen and testosterone have been found to influence drug enzyme activity in the CYP450 family – for example, enzyme CYP3A4 (phase I) is known to be up to 50% more active in women than men. Also, the enzyme CYP2B6 is involved in the metabolism of sertraline, a drug that is used in the treatment of depression. The activity of this enzyme is influenced by oestrogen and as a result women may metabolise sertraline more slowly, leading to higher concentrations in the body.

Other phase I enzymes also show sex-related differences. The gastric enzymes alcohol dehydrogenase and aldehyde dehydrogenase are phase I enzymes that metabolise alcohol. They are significantly more active in men than women. This results in a much higher bioavailability of alcohol in women and explains why men tend to cope better with alcohol than women.

Also, phase II conjugation enzymes display a lower activity in women than men.

## Ethnicity

Ethnicity can also play a role in differences in drug metabolism for an individual. Specifically, these variances have been attributed to genetic differences between ethnic groups. For example, some studies show that people of Asian and European descent have different genetic variants for CYP2C19 enzyme which can affect the metabolism of certain drugs (Zhong et al., 2017).

Furthermore, Black populations have a higher rate of a genetic variant that codes the CYP2D6 enzyme and reduces its activity (Rajman et al., 2017). These observations are clinically significant as CYP2D6 is responsible for the metabolism of a substantial number of drugs (approximately 20%). This further supports the argument for more individualised genomic assessment for drugs.

## Pregnancy

Liver enzyme activity fluctuates throughout pregnancy. For example, CYP1A2 activity is decreased during pregnancy, which may affect the metabolism of caffeine and theophylline (a bronchodilator that is used to prevent wheeziness, chest tightness and difficulty in breathing in asthma).

Conversely, activity of other enzymes (e.g. CYP2C9 and CYP3A) may increase during pregnancy, usually in the second and third trimesters. The activity of other enzymes, such as CYP2D6, varies throughout the pregnancy and may change from trimester to trimester. As CYP2D6 is a significant enzyme that metabolises many drugs, caution needs to be taken when prescribing or administering medication during pregnancy as there may be different responses to the same drugs taken during the same pregnancy.

## Environmental Factors

Exposure to pollutants in the environment can produce significant effects on drug metabolism. A common example of this is hydrocarbons in cigarette smoke which induce the activity of human cytochromes CYP1A2 and CYP2B6. These enzymes metabolise several clinically important drugs and therefore smoking can interfere with the metabolism of these drugs. Drug–drug interactions will be explored in depth later in this chapter.

## Disease

Drug metabolism will be impacted by disease. Any disease that impacts hepatic function will affect drug metabolism or biotransformation as the liver is the main site of metabolism. This includes conditions such as cirrhosis of the liver, malignancy and hepatitis. Any individual living with these conditions should be prescribed drugs cautiously to avoid elevated drug levels and toxicity, as their ability to metabolise a drug will be significantly impaired.

Cardiac disease can also affect the metabolism of drugs. Drug metabolism is dependent on drug delivery to the liver via the circulatory system. As blood flow is often compromised in cardiac disease, the extent to which a drug is transferred to the liver to undergo metabolism is reduced with the risk of increased drug levels and toxicity.

Thyroid hormones are essential in controlling the basal metabolic rate of the body and this affects drug metabolism. Hyperthyroidism can increase the rate of metabolism of some drugs and hypothyroidism can do the opposite. Other diseases such as diabetes, pulmonary conditions and endocrine deficiencies are believed to affect drug metabolism, but the mechanisms for these effects are not completely understood.

Individuals living with chronic diseases are often prescribed many drugs and therefore are more at risk of adverse reactions caused by drug–drug interactions that will either induce or inhibit enzyme actions. This will be explored in depth later in this chapter.

---

### PAUSE AND REFLECT 4.2

Age, sex, ethnicity, pregnancy, environmental factors and disease may all affect an individual's ability to metabolise drugs. Provide an example of how they impact the metabolism of drugs and, in each case, the considerations you need to take when caring for these individuals.

# CYP450 ENZYME INDUCTION AND ENZYME INHIBITION

The CYP450 enzyme system is potentially the source of drug–drug and drug–food interactions and therefore drug levels may be affected. These risk elevated drug levels and toxicity or drug levels which are below therapeutic range.

## CYP450 Enzyme Induction

The action of several of the isoenzymes within the CYP450 enzyme system may be induced by the co-administration of another drug or food. This means that more of the enzyme is produced over time resulting in rapid metabolism of the drug and a reduction in therapeutic levels (i.e. levels are **sub-therapeutic** and the action of the drug is reduced. Let us consider some examples.

The isoenzyme CYP1A2 acts on the metabolism of the anti-psychotic drug clozapine to prepare it for excretion. However, the aromatic hydrocarbons in cigarette smoke are an inducer of CYP1A2, which means that over time, more of these enzymes are produced. Clozapine will therefore be metabolised more rapidly resulting in lower therapeutic levels and poor management of the symptoms of psychosis.

Similarly, the herbal product St John's Wort, sold to relieve symptoms of depression, induces the CYP450 isoenzyme CYP3A4, which metabolises the contraceptive pill. Therefore, if St John's Wort and the contraceptive pill are taken concurrently, the contraceptive pill will be more rapidly metabolised, resulting in contraceptive failure.

---

### PAUSE AND REFLECT 4.3

Consider the role of herbal supplements in pharmacotherapy. Identify a herbal supplement and discuss its potential benefits and risks. How can patients ensure they are using herbal supplements safely and effectively?

---

## CYP Enzyme Inhibition

Drugs or foodstuffs when administered concurrently with a drug can result in enzyme inhibition. Enzyme inhibition results in less enzyme activity. This means that there is less of the isoenzyme CYP450 produced, which means the drug is not metabolised as expected and risks elevated drug levels and drug toxicity or overdose.

Drugs which are potent inhibitors of the isoenzyme CYP3A4 include ketoconazole, erythromycin and verapamil to name but a few. Some important CYP3A4 interactions may, however, occur in the intestines rather than the liver. This is seen with grapefruit juice.

To give examples:

- A common drug–drug interaction which involves the isoenzyme CYP3A4 involves the co-administration of clarithromycin and simvastatin. Simvastatin is metabolised by the isoenzyme CYP3A4. However, clarithromycin results in the inhibition of CYP3A4, with the result that simvastatin is not metabolised. There will be an increase in the drug levels of simvastatin resulting in myopathy or rhabdomyolysis (destruction of striated muscle cells).
- Verapamil inhibits the isoenzyme CYP3A4. When administered simultaneously with prednisone, the metabolism of prednisone is reduced, resulting in enhanced immunosuppression.
- Grapefruit juice, a powerful inhibitor of the isoenzyme CYP3A4 can result in increased levels of the antihypertensive drug nifedipine. This will cause significant hypotension.
- The action of disulfiram as an enzyme inhibitor is prescribed to manage the metabolism of alcohol and is a diversion therapy for those who are alcohol dependent. In normal circumstances the liver metabolises alcohol to produce acetaldehyde using the enzyme alcohol dehydrogenase. The enzyme aldehyde dehydrogenase and CYP2E1, found in the liver and the brain, further oxidise acetaldehyde to acetic acid in preparation for excretion. Disulfiram is an inhibitor of CYP2E1, which means that excess acetaldehyde remains in the body, which causes significant, adverse and unpleasant effects when alcohol is consumed.

Table 4.2 gives further examples of enzyme inhibition and induction.

**Table 4.2** Drugs affecting the action of cytochrome P450 enzymes

**Drugs affecting the action of cytochrome P450 enzymes**
(not an exhaustive list)

| CYP450 isoenzyme | Enzyme inducer | Enzyme inhibitor |
|---|---|---|
| CYP1A2 | cigarette smoke | ciprofloxacin |
|  | carbamazepine | fluvoxamine |
| CYP3A4/CYP3A5 | nevirapine, phenobarbital, rifampicin, St John's wort | ciprofloxacin |
|  |  | clarithromycin |
|  |  | erythromycin |
|  |  | fluconazole |
|  |  | ketoconazole |
|  |  | diltiazem |
|  |  | grapefruit juice |
|  |  | verapamil |
|  |  | ritonavir |
| CYP2C8 | rifampicin | clopidogrel |
|  |  | trimethoprim |

| | | |
|---|---|---|
| CYP2C9 | carbamazepine, St John's Wort | amiodarone, fluconazole, metronidazole |
| CYP2C19 | St John's Wort | fluvoxamine, ketoconazole, ticlopidine |
| CYP2B6 | rifampicin | ticlopidine |
| CYP2E1 | ethanol, isoniazid | disulfiram |

Other clinically relevant complications can occur when drugs employ the same metabolic pathways and therefore 'compete' for the same active site on the metabolising enzyme. For example, alcohol and phenobarbitone, a drug prescribed for sedation and status epilepticus utilise CYP2E1. If alcohol and phenobarbitone are administered together, the active sites of the CYP2E1 enzymes are 'taken up' in the metabolism of alcohol, resulting in the phenobarbitone not being adequately metabolised. The synergistic effects of alcohol and phenobarbitone will result in excessive sedation and toxicity.

## Entero-Hepatic Recycling

There are occasions when the chemical property of the drug is such that it leaves the liver and enters the biliary system. The liver is responsible for the production of bile, which is stored in the gall bladder and enters the small intestine via the bile duct. Lipophilic drug molecules present in the bile will then re-enter the small intestine and be reabsorbed for a second time. This process will inevitably extend the half-life of a drug and prolong its action. Drugs which undergo extensive **entero-hepatic recycling** include diazepam and lorazepam (see Figure 4.5).

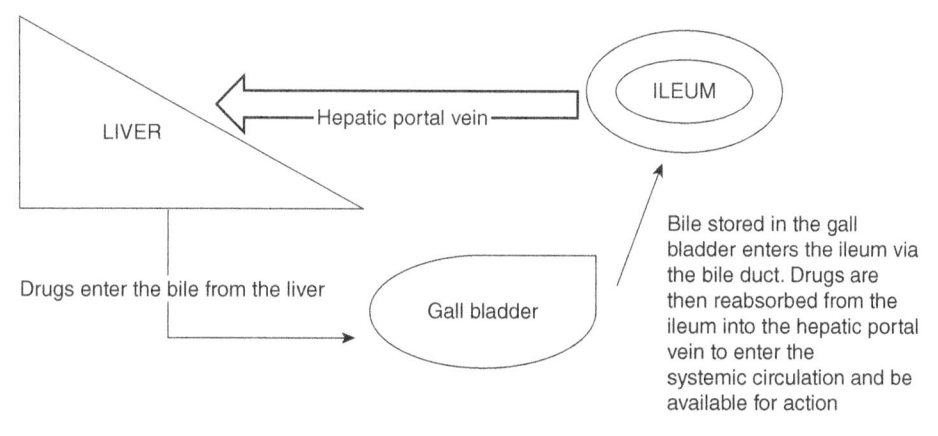

**Figure 4.5** Entero-hepatic recycling

## Half-Life of a Drug

The rate of drug absorption and excretion determines the half-life of a drug, which is recorded in time and is an important pharmacokinetic principle. Before exploring half-life (abbreviated to 't½' sometimes) a simple definition is: 'Half-life is the time it takes for the concentration (or amount) of a drug in a person's body to decrease by half.'

The half-life of a drug is largely set by how long the body takes to metabolise and/or eliminate the drug from the body. Without knowing much more about this concept than these two facts, there are several facts which need to be appreciated about the concept of half-life. From the pharmacological perspective the concept of the half-life of a drug has many applications. It allows us to set the dose interval for the drug. From the simple definition above, it is easy to see that drugs with short half-lives need more frequent dosing. It can also dictate the route of administration, so whilst the half-life of most drugs can be measured in hours, for some drugs the half-life can be measured in seconds. In these cases, it is easy to speculate that the oral route of administration of drugs with very short half-lives in the region of seconds might not be suitable for oral administration. Looking at some drug examples, it is easy to see that only the intravenous route would be suitable.

- *Adenosine (t½ = 10 seconds)*: Adenosine is a medication used to treat certain irregular cardiac rhythms. It has a short half-life, in seconds, and is typically administered as a rapid intravenous injection.
- *Dobutamine (t½ = 2–5 minutes)*: Dobutamine is a medication used to increase heart rate and improve cardiac output in conditions like cardiac failure. It has a short half-life and is administered intravenously.

At first glance it might appear that this is an inconvenience and increases the risk of intravenous complications rather than adopting the oral route. However, by understanding the concept of half-life and in competent hands, the short half-life of these drugs is of clinical benefit. For example, the short half-life of adenosine is one of the reasons it is effective in rapidly slowing down the heart rate and restoring normal rhythm in certain cardiac conditions. Drugs with short half-lives rapidly reach therapeutic levels and so can have a rapid effect. In the case of dobutamine, the short half-life allows healthcare providers to adjust the dosage and titrate the drug to achieve the desired cardiac response while considering its rapid elimination from the body. In both cases, when the drug is stopped it only takes a very short time (minutes) to reach levels that no longer have a clinical effect, so once the immediate critical period is over it makes it easier to transfer to a more long-term treatment without too much delay and crossover.

Here are some other examples of drugs with short half-lives:

- *Nitroprusside* is a vasodilator used to treat **hypertensive** emergencies. It has a short half-life and is typically administered intravenously.

- *Milrinone* is a medication used to increase heart contraction and improve cardiac output. It has a short half-life and is administered intravenously.
- *Sodium thiopental* is a barbiturate anaesthetic rather than a drug used for therapeutic purposes but it has a very short half-life, typically measured in minutes.

Understanding the half-life of a drug can inform us whether alternative formulations would be helpful. A classic example is morphine. Its half-life is not that short, at around three hours. Depending on what it is being used for, this shorter half-life can be a clinical problem. It is easy to see that this half-life wouldn't be a problem as a one-off dose to relieve pain during a brief acute episode of pain but in other cases, such as in palliative care, the need for repeated doses to maintain therapeutic levels is inconvenient and risks poor analgesic control. The understanding of half-life in this case led to the recognition, and supported the formulation of, modified release formulations of morphine.

Although dose intervals are outlined in guidance and documentation, individual patient factors cannot be ignored. This is because patient factors can influence the half-life of a drug and it is important to monitor for physiological factors that would alter half-life, so that they can be considered when administering drugs to patients to prevent accumulation and toxicity. For example, atenolol is a beta-blocker used to treat conditions such as hypertension and certain cardiac-related conditions and is eliminated unchanged by renal excretion. The half-life of atenolol in individuals with normal kidney function is typically around six to seven hours. In patients with poor renal function, the elimination of certain drugs, including atenolol, can be impaired. When kidney function is compromised, the clearance of renally excreted drugs from the body can be reduced, leading to an increase in their half-life. This means that atenolol remains in the body for a longer period before it is eliminated, accumulating and potentially increasing the risk of adverse effects such as bradycardia.

Prescribers often need to adjust the dosage and administration of drugs like atenolol in patients with impaired renal function to avoid potential complications. This might involve reducing the dose, increasing the dosing interval or choosing alternative medications that are better tolerated in individuals with renal impairment.

Finally, an appreciation of the concept of the half-life of a drug can help understand some common issues that are encountered in clinical practice, and this can determine how a drug is best used. Take naloxone for instance. Naloxone is a medication commonly used as an opioid receptor antagonist to rapidly reverse the effects of opioid overdose. When administered, naloxone binds to opioid receptors in the brain and blocks the effects of opioids, effectively reversing respiratory depression and other life-threatening symptoms associated with opioid overdose, often amongst people using drugs such as diamorphine (heroin) illicitly. At this point the short half-life works in our favour as it can rapidly reach therapeutic levels. However, since naloxone has a relatively short half-life (around 30–80 minutes) compared to the activity of diamorphine which can be hours, its effects on opioid receptors can wear off relatively quickly and, more importantly, whilst there is still plenty of opioid active in the person's body. This can mean that respiratory depression/arrest returns. It is important to monitor patients closely and has led to practices such as the administration of intranasal or intravenously administered naloxone with an intramuscular injection which then gradually enters systemic circulation providing a reservoir of naloxone over a longer period.

This last example is a good illustration of a point to remain aware of when reading about the half-lives of drugs. Search for details of the half-life of diamorphine and you will probably find that it is relatively short, usually ranging from about two to six minutes. In fact, this is the key to one reason why it is so addictive: it gives an extremely fast high and then a very rapid withdrawal and provokes the need for repeated doses to maintain its effects, which can lead to a cycle of tolerance, dependence and addiction. This short half-life seems to be at odds with the example given. However, it's important to note that diamorphine is rapidly metabolised in the body into its active metabolite 6-monoacetylmorphine (6-MAM), and then further metabolised into morphine. As a result, the effects of diamorphine are often short-lived, but it is quickly converted into molecules or drugs with longer half-lives that have the same effect.

To add a little more depth to our understanding of half-life using some visual representations, let's look at a couple more examples. There is a concept that after four or five half-lives a drug can be considered to have been eliminated from the body entirely, so any actual drug levels at this point are not going to be clinically significant (see Figure 4.6).

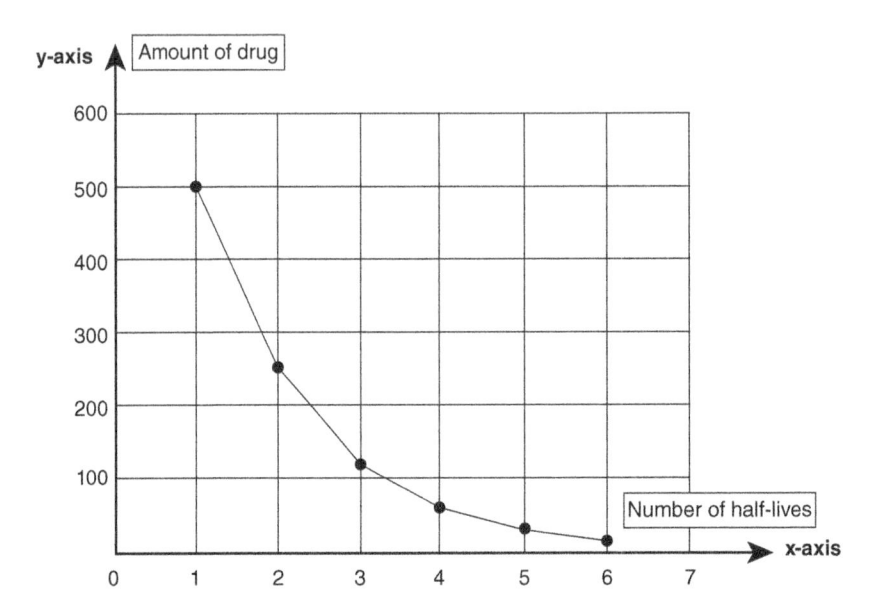

**Figure 4.6** Pharmacology half-life exponential decay

On the x-axis you can see the half-life noted as one half-life, two half-lives and so on, and on the y-axis, the drug level. Now, whatever numbers you put in realistically, you will see that the amount of drug remaining after five half-lives is so small it won't be having a clinical effect unless of course there are active metabolites in which case the illustration would need to continue with these.

Let's take the example of amiodarone. This is another drug used to treat cardiac arrythmia, like adenosine, but in this case, amiodarone has a very long half-life of 50 days. The therapeutic range for amiodarone is typically 2.5 micrograms per millilitre down to 0.8 micrograms per millilitre depending on the type of arrythmia. Here is a calculation, if we assume someone has had levels of 2.5 micrograms per millilitre and then the drug is stopped after 50 days the drugs levels could be estimated at 1.25 micrograms per millilitre, still well within the therapeutic range. In fact, if we take the next half-life drop, at 100 days, the drug level would be half of what it was at 50 days and be 0.625 micrograms per millilitre. Now below the therapeutic range, but this would mean the drug would have still been having an effect for around three months without taking any further medication. This could be a real problem if a change of medication was required due to a patient experiencing adverse effects.

Looking at this example, it can be interesting to think about the half-lives of common drugs and how these affect their use in practice, such as dosing intervals, the duration of therapeutic effects, or its specific therapeutic role. Table 4.3 provides some examples of the half-life of drugs (in hours).

**Table 4.3** Examples of the half-life of drugs

| Drug | Half-life/hours |
| --- | --- |
| diazepam | 43 |
| digoxin | 39 |
| fluoxetine | 53 |
| lithium | 22 |
| midazolam | 1.9 |
| warfarin | 37 |

### PAUSE AND REFLECT 4.4

Think about the concept of drug half-life. Identify at least three medications you know and research their half-lives. How does the half-life of each drug influence its dosing schedule?

## Prodrugs

A prodrug is a drug that is not pharmacologically active until it has undergone some form of conversion in the body. For most drugs in clinical practice this will be through metabolism by the liver.

The fact that the liver is necessary to convert the inactive drug into a drug that has the pharmacological effect logically suggests that these drugs would be given in their oral form rather than by injection, taking advantage of first-pass metabolism. The list of prodrugs below cross-referenced against the British National Formulary (BNF) or the Electronic Medicines Compendium (EMC) confirms this.

Here is a list of some well-known prodrugs:

- *Codeine*: Converts to morphine in the body
- *Enalapril*: Converts to enalaprilat, an **angiotensin-converting enzyme (ACE) inhibitor**
- *Clopidogrel*: Converts to its active form in the body, inhibiting platelet aggregation
- *Oseltamivir*: Converts to its active form, oseltamivir carboxylate, which inhibits neuraminidase in influenza viruses
- *Valacyclovir*: Converts to acyclovir, an antiviral used to treat herpes infections
- *Lisdexamfetamine*: Converts to dextroamphetamine in the body, used to treat attention deficit hyperactivity disorder (ADHD)
- *Fosamprenavir*: Converts to amprenavir, an antiretroviral used in HIV treatment
- *Prednisone*: Converts to prednisolone, a corticosteroid with anti-inflammatory properties
- *Captopril*: Converts to captopril disulfide, an angiotensin-converting enzyme (ACE) inhibitor

In general, there would be no major advantage in administering or taking these drugs by a parenteral route because they would not become active until they had been metabolised. Since parenteral routes are used either for rapid action or when other routes are not clinically acceptable, it would make sense to use non-prodrugs for the intravenous route most of the time.

The question would be, why use a prodrug at all? Sometimes there is no good reason for this and it is just a consequence of the drug having been developed, and just happening to be a prodrug. But more often the reason to develop a prodrug is to enhance drug delivery, solubility, absorption or to minimise adverse effects.

For example, the angiotensin-converting enzyme inhibitors (ACEIs) that were first developed were very successful from a pharmacodynamic perspective in that they had a profound ability to reduce blood pressure. However, their bioavailability was very poor and so they needed to be given in larger doses due to their poor absorption. Large doses cost more money and unabsorbed medications can increase adverse gastrointestinal effects. The most common ACEIs today are prodrugs, such as ramipril, that can be given in smaller doses and have higher bioavailability.

It is still necessary, however, to keep some ACEIs that are not prodrugs, perhaps those with the best bioavailability in their class or whose molecule has been adjusted not to be a prodrug but are better absorbed. Imagine, for example, a patient with variable liver function. This could be because they have cardiac failure and so each day the amount of blood flow around the body that their heart can provide varies and this can affect the function of various other organs including the liver. In these cases, a clinician may opt for an ACEI like lisinopril which is a not a prodrug. Lisinopril is administered in its active form and directly exerts its therapeutic effects without needing to be metabolically activated. For this reason it is not reliant on the metabolising capacity of the liver and should lead to a more consistent effect on the patient.

So far, these have been examples of prodrugs that have been developed to increase bioavailability to reduce costs and adverse effects or are prodrugs simply by chance arising from their development. But there is one more good set of examples related to safety. An example would be the prodrug cyclophosphamide. Cyclophosphamide is an alkylating agent commonly used in chemotherapy to treat various types of cancers, including leukaemia, lymphoma and solid tumours. It is designed as a prodrug to improve its therapeutic efficacy and reduce its toxicity. Cyclophosphamide is administered in its inactive form. Once inside the body, it undergoes metabolic activation by the liver's enzymes, mainly the cytochrome P450 system, to form its active metabolites, including phosphoramide mustard and acrolein. These active metabolites are responsible for the anti-cancer effects of cyclophosphamide. Phosphoramide mustard binds to DNA and interferes with its replication and transcription, leading to cell death, while acrolein contributes to the drug's toxic side effects, particularly those affecting the urinary system. This prodrug design allows for a controlled release of the active compounds within the body, increasing the drug's **selectivity** for cancer cells and reducing damage to healthy tissues.

---

### PAUSE AND REFLECT 4.5

Reflect on the role of prodrugs in pharmacology. Identify a prodrug and describe how it is activated in the body. What are the advantages of using a prodrug over the active form of the drug?

---

## THERAPEUTIC WINDOW AND THERAPEUTIC INDEX

A drug's half-life, determined by the rate and extent of absorption, metabolism and excretion will affect drug levels in the body. For drugs which are administered on a frequent basis to manage chronic conditions or prevent ill health, the drug levels need to achieve a 'steady state' in that levels are both safe and therapeutic. It is generally accepted that it takes five times a drug's half-life to maintain a steady state when administered frequently. For example, if the half-life of morphine sulphate is four hours, it takes approximately 20 hours of frequent dosing to achieve a steady state and maintain the analgesic effect.

The graph in Figure 4.7 shows the extent of the 'therapeutic window' to ensure that the plasma drug concentration is neither too high, resulting in adverse drug reactions and toxicity, nor too low, where therapeutic effect is not achieved. When a drug is administered, for example every four hours over a period, the dose and the frequency administered must ensure the drug levels are therapeutic.

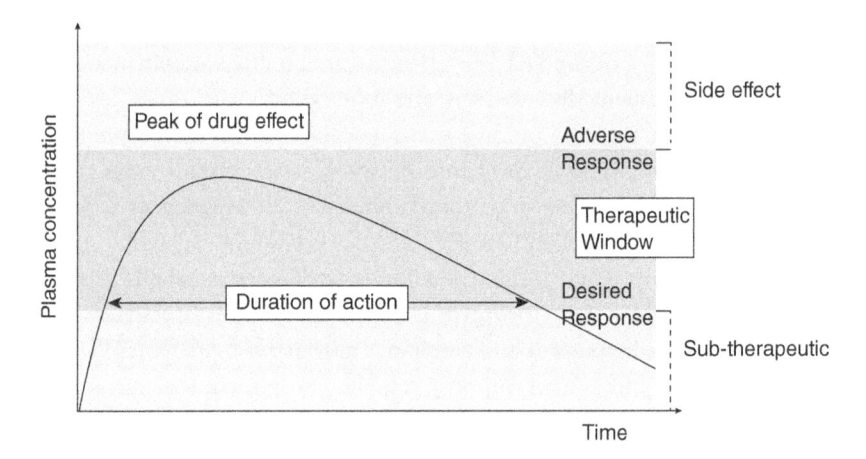

**Figure 4.7** The extent of the 'therapeutic window'

The *therapeutic index* (TI), also referred to as the *therapeutic ratio* of a drug, is a numerical value which is representative of a drug's safety profile. In animal models (not human clinical trials), the dose which would be fatal in 50% of the human population is designated $LD_{50}$ (median lethal dose) and the dose that would be minimally effective in 50% of the population is designated $ED_{50}$ (median effective dose). The lethal dose of a drug for 50% of the population $LD_{50}$ is then divided by the minimum effective dose $ED_{50}$ for 50% of the population. This gives us the figure for the TI. To give an example, if the $LD_{50}$ is 10 mg and the $ED_{50}$ is 5 mg, the TI is calculated as 2:

$$\text{Therapeutic Index} = \frac{LD_{50}}{ED_{50}}$$

In clinical settings, it is the toxic dose (TD) which is recorded and not the lethal dose (LD). A toxic dose refers to the amount of a drug or substance that causes harmful effects or toxicity in the body, exceeding the level considered safe for therapeutic use.

Drugs with a high TI, considered to be greater than 10, are deemed safer because the difference between the TD and ED is significant.

For drugs with a low TI or narrow therapeutic range (e.g. lithium carbonate, TI = 2; digoxin, TI = 2; theophylline, TI = 1.5; and warfarin, TI = 2.5), it is important that drug levels are regularly monitored to prevent the risk of drug toxicity.

> **PAUSE AND REFLECT 4.6**
>
> How does knowledge and understanding of the therapeutic window of a drug influence its dosage and patient safety?
>
> Can you think of any drugs for which drug levels must be monitored? Consider the reasons for this in relation to patient safety.

## CHAPTER SUMMARY

Chapter 4 has examined the third stage of pharmacokinetics: drug metabolism. The physiology of the liver is described with a particular focus on the role and action of the CYP450 enzyme system in drug metabolism. Several important factors are explored which may affect the rate and extent of drug metabolism and ultimately drug levels. Key pharmacokinetic concepts – a drug's half-life, therapeutic window, therapeutic index and entero-hepatic recycling are explained in relation to the safe and therapeutic administration and monitoring of drugs.

# DRUG EXCRETION 5

---
### LEARNING OUTCOMES
---

By the end of this chapter, you should be able to:

1. Explain renal anatomy and physiology relevant to drug elimination
2. Discuss the different routes of drug excretion
3. Discuss 'clearance rates' and impact on a drug's half-life
4. Discuss the factors that influence the excretion of drugs and medicine therapeutics

---

## INTRODUCTION

This chapter explores the fourth and final stage of the pharmacokinetic process, drug excretion (clearance or elimination).

Excretion is defined as the irreversible removal of drugs from the body, either as a metabolite or unchanged drug. There are many different routes of excretion, the most significant being via urine, and the kidneys play a vital role in this. On average, the kidneys filter 200 L a day from the renal blood flow, facilitating the excretion of toxins, waste products and ions from the body whilst keeping essential substances in the blood.

## ANATOMY OF THE KIDNEYS

The kidneys are reddish-brown bean-shaped organs found behind the parietal peritoneum, against the deep back muscles. They are enclosed in a tough and fibrous capsule.

The kidneys are organised into two main regions: the **outer renal cortex** and the **inner renal medulla**. The cortex extends into the medulla, dividing it into triangular shapes – these are known as renal pyramids. The top of a renal pyramid is called a renal papilla. Each renal papilla is associated with a structure known as the minor calyx, which collects urine from the pyramids. The minor calices combine to create a major calyx. Urine passes through the major calices into the renal pelvis, a flattened and funnel-shaped structure. From the renal pelvis, urine drains into the ureter, which transports it to the bladder for storage (see Figure 5.1).

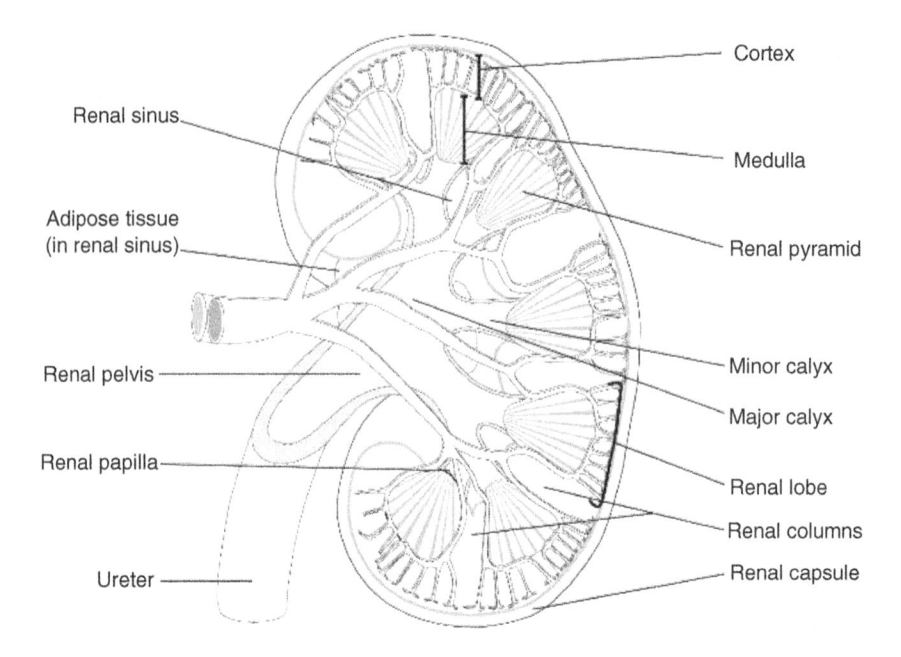

**Figure 5.1** The kidney

The kidneys are continuously supplied with blood from the renal arteries, which stems from the abdominal aorta and transports large blood volumes. The kidneys are drained of venous blood by renal veins, which empty directly into the vena cava (see Figure 5.2).

The kidney contains about one million nephrons, mainly in the cortex. Nephrons are the functional units of the kidney and contain a renal corpuscle and a renal tubule. The renal corpuscle consists of the Bowman's capsule and a network of capillaries called the glomerulus.

The renal tubule is a long tube that can be divided into three sections: the proximal convoluted tubule, nephron loop (loop of Henle) and distal convoluted loop (see Figure 5.3).

Excretion is defined as the irreversible removal of drugs from the body and the kidney is the main organ involved in excretion. The kidneys filter toxins, waste products and ions from approximately 200 L of fluid, whilst keeping essential substances in the blood.

They produce urine in three important stages: *glomerular filtration, tubular reabsorption* and *tubular excretion.*

The purpose of urine is to remove excess water and metabolic waste from the body. It also plays an important role in controlling blood pressure, electrolyte balance and overall fluid levels.

DRUG EXCRETION | 103

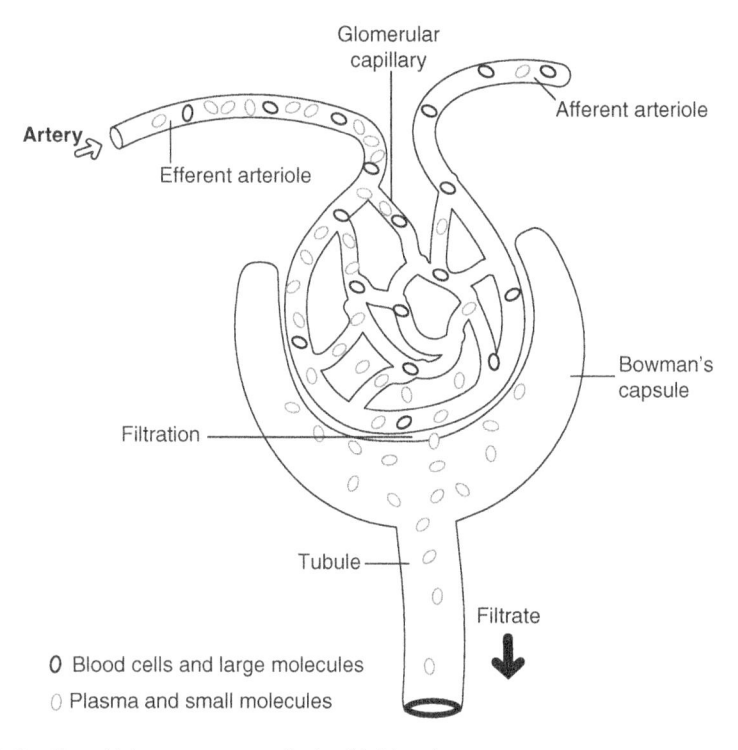

**Figure 5.2** How kidneys are supplied with blood

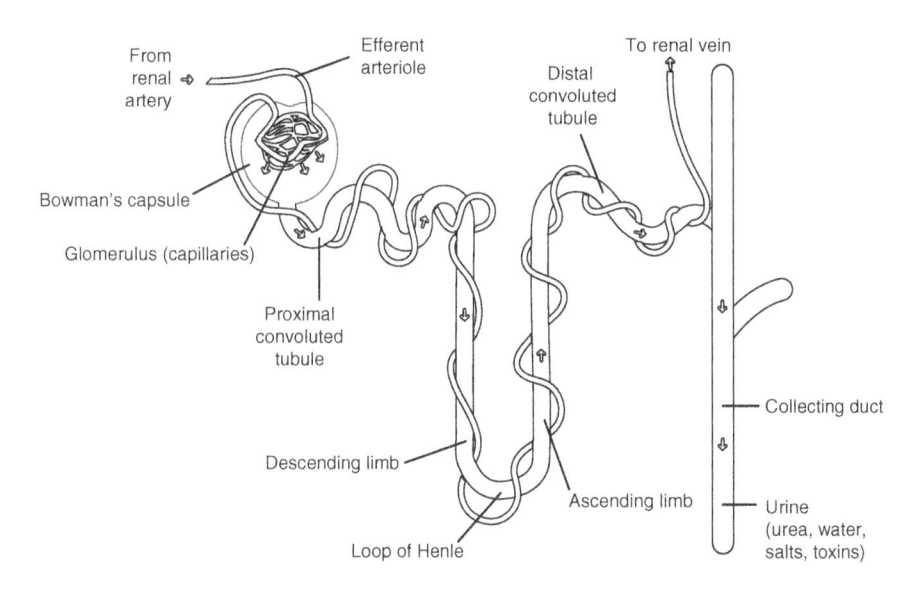

**Figure 5.3** The renal tubule

## Glomerular Filtration

Filtration takes place in the semi-permeable walls of the glomerulus and glomerular capsule. The glomerulus contains a network of capillaries. Blood flows through these capillaries and with the aid of hydrostatic pressures, components of the blood are filtered through an ultrafiltration barrier into the glomerular capsule. The ultrafiltration barrier allows water, and anything dissolved in it (including water-soluble drugs) and small particles to pass through it. However, it prevents larger particles such as blood cells and plasma proteins from passing. Therefore, any plasma-bound drugs cannot pass through and remain in the circulation, but free or unbound drugs will. The fluid in the glomerular (Bowman's) capsule is known as filtrate and drains directly into the proximal tubule of the nephron.

The glomerular filtration rate (GFR) is the amount of filtrate created per minute by all nephrons in both kidneys. The GFR is a good indicator of how well the kidneys are working.

## Tubular (selective) Reabsorption

Once the filtrate reaches the renal tubules and collecting ducts, reabsorption begins. Substances from the filtrate are selectively reabsorbed into the bloodstream. All glucose and amino acids as well as most of the water, sodium and other electrolytes are reabsorbed. Approximately 99% of what we filter is reabsorbed into the bloodstream. What is left over becomes urine (1% of the volume of the filtrate). We do not want drugs to be reabsorbed. Most drugs that have been metabolised by the liver are polar and this helps prevent reabsorption.

The pH of urine can either inhibit or enhance drug reabsorption in the renal tubule and in certain clinical situations we will manipulate the pH of urine to control the excretion of drugs and increase **renal clearance** of drugs. Most drugs are either weak acids or weak bases. Acidic drugs are more easily ionised in alkaline urine whilst alkaline drugs are more easily ionised in acidic urine. Ionised (or polar) substances, which are more water soluble, will be more readily excreted. This is important when an individual takes an overdose of acetylsalicylic acid (aspirin). By providing an infusion of sodium bicarbonate, the urine will become more alkaline, increasing the ionisation of salicylic acid (metabolite of aspirin) and therefore it will be excreted more quickly from the body.

## Tubular Secretion

Tubular secretion selectively moves substances from the blood into the renal tubule to be excreted. It disposes of substances such as drugs, particularly those that are bound to plasma proteins. This is because proteins are not filtered and neither are the substances bound to them, so they need to be secreted. Tubular secretion also eliminates undesirable substances such as urea. It removes excessive potassium ions from the body. All potassium ions are reabsorbed from the filtrate in the proximal tubule, so all potassium in the urine comes from tubular secretion at the end of the distal convoluted tubule. Tubular secretion is also involved in controlling the blood pH by secreting hydrogen ions.

Urine is the product of glomerular filtration, tubular reabsorption and tubular secretion. It drains from the tubules into the renal pelvis and then onto the ureters. From here it is taken to the bladder where it is stored until micturition. We produce between 0.6 L and 2 L of urine a day and its composition can be an important indicator of disease or illness. Testing of urine (urinalysis) for abnormal substances can lead to a diagnosis of underlying pathologies.

## DRUG CLEARANCE

Drug clearance refers to the volume of plasma cleared of a drug over a specified time. Drug clearance considers hepatic, renal and other modes of clearance. However, as drug excretion takes place mainly via the urine, renal function will directly impact how much a drug is cleared from the body.

From a pharmacological and toxicological perspective, the main function of the liver is to inactivate toxins either before they have reached systemic circulation, by first-pass metabolism, or reduce continued exposure through metabolism. However, sometimes the liver does not have the metabolic enzymes required to deal with certain molecules and so some drugs cannot be metabolised or transformed in any way by the liver. For the most part, elimination of these types of drugs, most of which are relatively water soluble, is by renal excretion.

The kidneys are therefore a vital route to drug clearance and elimination. This can be for those drugs that cannot be metabolised by the liver, or it can also be for relatively water soluble, polar metabolites which do not need further metabolism because they are inactive or active or toxic metabolites that cannot be metabolised by the liver any further.

It can be seen then that the kidney is important in drugs which cannot be metabolised by the liver or have renally excreted active or toxic metabolites and that adequate renal function is key to successful elimination. There are several groups for whom these categories of drug or metabolites would be problematic (e.g elderly people, neonates or those with poor renal function). It is important to remember that renal excretion is just one aspect of a drug's pharmacokinetics, and factors such as metabolism, protein binding and other elimination pathways can also contribute to a drug's overall clearance from the body. Often dose adjustments may be necessary for individuals with impaired kidney function to prevent drug accumulation and potential adverse effects.

The following are examples of drugs which are primarily or only renally excreted:

- *Lithium* is commonly used to treat bipolar disorder. It has a narrow therapeutic window, and its elimination occurs mainly through the kidneys. Monitoring serum lithium levels is crucial to avoid toxicity.
- *Aminoglycoside antibiotics* (e.g. gentamicin, tobramycin) are a class of antibiotics used to treat serious bacterial infections. They are known for their nephrotoxicity and ototoxicity. These drugs are almost entirely eliminated through renal excretion.

- *Ciprofloxacin* is a fluoroquinolone antibiotic. It is excreted primarily through the kidneys and is commonly used to treat various infections, including urinary tract infections.
- *Vancomycin* is an antibiotic used to treat infections caused by gram-positive bacteria. It has limited oral absorption and is typically administered intravenously. Its elimination is mainly through renal excretion.
- *Dabigatran* is an anticoagulant used to prevent stroke and blood clots. It is eliminated predominantly through the kidneys. Dosage adjustments are required for patients with impaired renal function to prevent excessive anticoagulation.
- *Methotrexate* is a chemotherapy drug used to treat various types of cancer and autoimmune diseases. It is primarily eliminated through renal excretion. Renal function monitoring is crucial to prevent toxicity.
- *Metformin* is an antidiabetic medication. It is primarily eliminated unchanged in the urine, and baseline renal function and ongoing monitoring are required to avoid the risk of accumulation in the body resulting in lactic acidosis.
- *Trimethoprim* is an antibiotic commonly used in urine infections.
- *Mefenamic acid* is a non-steroidal anti-inflammatory drug (NSAID) used for pain relief. It is primarily excreted through the kidneys, and its elimination can be affected by renal function. This is especially problematic as NSAIDs can affect renal clearance themselves through prostaglandin inhibition.

Here are a few examples of drugs whose active or toxic metabolites are primarily or only renally excreted.

- *Morphine and morphine-6-glucuronide*: Morphine is metabolised into morphine-6-glucuronide, which is a more potent analgesic compound. Both morphine and its metabolite are primarily excreted through the kidneys. Accumulation of morphine-6-glucuronide can occur in patients with renal impairment, leading to increased analgesic effects and potential toxicity.
- *Hydromorphone and hydromorphone-3-glucuronide*: Like morphine, hydromorphone is metabolised into hydromorphone-3-glucuronide, which is also an active metabolite. Both the parent drug and its metabolite are renally excreted.
- *Quinidine, an anti-arrhythmic medication, and its active metabolite, 3-hydroxyquinidine*: Both quinidine and its metabolite are primarily excreted through the kidneys.

Now that there is an understanding that some molecules that are pharmacologically active are reliant on the kidney for elimination, some observations can be made and some more detailed examples can be given.

An initial and perhaps surprising observation is that sometimes it is important that a drug is *not* primarily metabolised by the body before being eliminated from systemic circulation. However, if we take the examples of the antibiotics ciprofloxacin and trimethoprim (nitrofurantoin too), they would be of no use if they were inactivated by the liver because these drugs need to be active at the point of the infection, which is in the bladder. And in fact, these drugs achieve high concentration in the urinary tract, making them effective for treating urinary tract infections (UTIs) caused by susceptible bacteria. Finally, though, it's worth noting that these drugs can be contraindicated (nitrofurantoin) or cautioned (ciprofloxacin, trimethoprim) in patients with significant renal impairment, as reduced kidney function can lead to the drug's accumulation and potential toxicity (for details look at the drug-specific product characteristics or refer to the latest guidance in the British National Formulary (BNF)).

Drugs that are renally excreted are likely to be relatively water soluble and so reach high concentrations in areas of the body that are associated with high concentration of fluids. For example, gentamicin is a drug with a narrow therapeutic window; there is not much difference between the dose required to treat versus the dose that will harm. As it is highly water soluble and is eliminated unchanged by the renal route it will be more concentrated in the kidney and so more likely to damage this organ than others. Additionally, gentamicin can cause ototoxicity by damaging the nerves in the fluid-filled cochlea; again due to its polar nature it can be concentrated in this organ more than elsewhere in the body.

There are several drugs that are relatively lower risk than gentamicin but are used to treat long-term conditions and so there is a need for ongoing monitoring of renal function or observation for signs that accumulation is occurring. An example from the list would be metformin. The risk of lactic acidosis is very rare where renal function is normal and standard doses are prescribed. However, patients will be taking these medicines long term and their renal function may decline, either through natural age-related changes or because their condition can itself lead to progression through the stages of chronic kidney disease (CKD). In these cases, the monitoring is to pick up if there is a sufficient change in renal function to warrant a review of the medication, and if action is required this could take the form of a dose reduction or a change of medication to one that is not so reliant on renal function for elimination.

Finally, drugs that are exclusively renally excreted can be subject to significant and potentially harmful drug interactions. As one example, lithium is renally excreted and has a narrow therapeutic window. This means a small change in systemic drug levels due to changes in excretion by the renal route could be enough to cause toxicity. A good illustration of this would be the risk of taking NSAIDs with lithium. NSAIDs work by inhibiting prostaglandin synthesis, which is how they reduce inflammation. However, NSAIDs are non-selective and, whilst they are an essential drug to treat inflammatory conditions such as arthritis, the drug also affects prostaglandin synthesis in other parts of the body that rely on prostaglandins for normal function. In the case of the kidney, prostaglandins are essential to keep the renal tubules patent. In most cases the reduction in patency they cause is small and of no significance. However, when taking lithium, sufficient accumulation could occur due to reduced renal function caused by the NSAID, potentially leading to toxicity. This could be made even worse if the patient was also elderly as renal function always declines with age, or even dehydrated to the point that their renal function had become affected.

## IN SUMMARY

- *Several medications are predominantly eliminated through the kidneys via urine.* Inadequate renal function may result in decreased drug clearance, which may contribute to drug accumulation and an increased risk of adverse effects.
- *Renal clearance is comprised of filtration, secretion and reabsorption of medications in the kidneys.* Secretion actively transports drugs from blood to urine, and reabsorption can occur when drugs are reabsorbed back into the circulation from the urine.
- *Patients with diminished renal function may require lower doses or extended dosing intervals.* This is because impaired kidneys may not clear the drug effectively, resulting in protracted exposure and an increased risk of toxicity.
- *In patients with impaired renal function, drugs primarily eliminated by the kidneys may accumulate in the body.* This accumulation may result in heightened drug effects, potential organ damage and other adverse reactions.
- *Some pharmaceuticals are metabolised into active or toxic compounds, which are then excreted via the kidneys.* These metabolites can accumulate in patients with impaired renal function, compromising drug efficacy and safety.
- *Regular monitoring of renal function, typically by assessing glomerular filtration rate (GFR), is essential when prescribing drugs predominantly excreted by the kidneys.* Depending on the patient's renal function, dosage adjustments or medication substitutions may be necessary.
- *Monitoring renal function is particularly important in certain populations, such as elderly individuals and those with renal disease, where impaired function can affect drug clearance.* In children, the developing renal system must also be considered when determining drug dosing and intervals.
- *Some drugs can induce kidney damage or exacerbate pre-existing kidney conditions.* Monitoring renal function is essential for early detection of adverse effects when using such medications.
- *Therapeutic drug monitoring, maintaining the correct blood concentration, is crucial for drugs with a narrow therapeutic index.* Monitoring renal function ensures that drug concentrations are within the effective and safe range.

Although there are other routes of excretion – of bile, sweat, saliva, tears, faeces, breast milk and exhaled air – they cannot replace the kidney route of excretion. If you lose your kidneys, your sweat glands cannot take over! However, there is clinical importance in some of the alternative routes of excretion.

---

### PAUSE AND REFLECT 5.1

For drugs excreted renally, how does renal failure affect drug levels, the half-life of a drug and drug safety?

## The Hepatobiliary System

Some drugs and drug metabolites are excreted by the hepatobiliary system. As the liver filters blood, some drugs (and their metabolites) are actively transported by liver cells (hepatocytes) to bile. Bile flows through the bile duct to the gall bladder and then to the intestines. From here the drug may be excreted in the faeces. However, some drugs are reabsorbed into the bloodstream and eventually return to the liver – this is the entero-hepatic cycle (see Chapter 4). Therefore, biliary excretion eliminates drugs from the body only to the degree that enterohepatic cycling is incomplete (i.e. when some of the excreted drug is not reabsorbed from the intestine and is eliminated through the faeces).

Factors which influence excretion by the biliary tract are often the properties of the drug such as polarity and molecular size. They are mainly lipophilic, large, and/or polar molecules. Conjugation also facilitates biliary excretion. Rifampicin – an antibiotic used in the treatment of tuberculosis – is conjugated in the liver to glucuronic acid and then excreted in the bile (and urine).

Drugs that are excreted by the hepatobiliary system may be affected by individual differences in biliary elimination or cholestatic and liver disease. Reduced bile flow may result in an increased risk of drug toxicity.

Conditions that cause decreased blood flow to the liver can also affect the metabolism and excretion of drugs. For example, conditions such as shock, hypovolemia or hypotension cause decreased liver perfusion and may require adjustment of dosages of medication.

## Exhaled Air

The process of removing drugs from the body via exhaled air is known as pulmonary excretion. This is the primary route for volatile anaesthetic gases (such as nitrous oxide) to be eliminated from the body. Volatile substances are those that can easily change from a liquid phase to a gas phase.

Drugs with high solubility in blood are more likely to be excreted through the lungs. This is an important protective measure, as demonstrated when we drink alcohol. Alcohol (or ethanol) is metabolised by the liver by an enzyme called alcohol dehydrogenase (ADH). As we drink more alcohol, there are not enough ADH molecules to metabolise it quickly enough and it begins to accumulate in the bloodstream, leading to an increase in blood alcohol concentration. The concentration of ethanol in the blood exceeds the concentration of ethanol in the alveoli (which is zero). Ethanol then diffuses into the air sacs until the concentration in blood relative to that in air achieves a constant ratio or equilibrium. The molecules of ethanol continue to move back and forth if this equilibrium is disturbed. So, when the ethanol is excreted in the breath, an equal amount of ethanol moves from the bloodstream to the alveoli. That is why breathalyser tests are used by the police to detect the amount of alcohol in an individual.

## Breast Milk

It is well documented that drugs ingested by the mother and/or their metabolites transfer to breast milk and therefore can be excreted via this route. Drugs with low molecular weight, low maternal plasma protein binding and high lipophilicity are more likely to transfer to breast milk. This is due to the properties of milk, including lower pH and higher lipid content in comparison to plasma. Also, milk compositions change over the weeks following birth from colostrum to mature milk and within the feed itself, between fore and hind milk. These factors contribute to the time-dependent variation of drug excretion into milk. There have been several pathways identified for how drugs transfer into milk, including active transport and carrier-mediated transport, but passive diffusion accounts for the majority of drug pathways.

Most drugs administered to the lactating mother appear in milk in concentrations similar to maternal plasma concentrations. This, alongside the functional immaturity of the liver and kidneys in neonates, raises concerns about the effect of any transferred drug on the child. The use of medications in breastfeeding mothers always requires an assessment of risk to the child versus the therapeutic benefit for the mother. The enormous benefits of breastfeeding are well known, but the risks of most medications used in breastfeeding should always be taken into consideration.

Sweat, saliva and tears are minor routes of drug excretion. Drugs that are excreted by these bodily fluids are lipophilic, pH dependent and transported via passive diffusion. Though not a particularly effective route of elimination, the consequences of excretion of drugs via these routes may be of interest. For example, excretion of the drug in tears could cause concern if it was rifampicin, which is bright red! Patients may think they are bleeding from their eyes or at least it could ruin someone's soft contact lenses if you don't warn them not to wear them whilst taking the drug!

Saliva is not truly an excretory route. However, as it is usually swallowed, this allows some drugs to be reabsorbed from the gastrointestinal tract. A bitter taste in the mouth can be an indicator that the drug has been excreted. Salivary concentration of lipid-soluble drugs reflects plasma concentration of the drug but is not always accurate. However, obtaining saliva samples is cheap, non-invasive and quick, so they are useful in detecting disease and drug abuse.

### PAUSE AND REFLECT 5.2

Choose several drugs that you are familiar with and for each, identify:

1. The primary route of excretion
2. The drug's half-life
3. Are they excreted 'changed' or 'unchanged'

## CHAPTER SUMMARY

Chapter 5 has explored the different routes of drug excretion, with a specific focus on the role of the renal system. Several factors affect the renal clearance of drugs, and these are considered with respect to ensuring that drug levels remain safe and therapeutic following administration.

# PRINCIPLES OF PHARMACODYNAMICS 6

---
### LEARNING OUTCOMES
---

By the end of this chapter, you should be able to:

1 Explain, using named examples, the following concepts relating to the mode of action of a drug: cellular transport systems: ligand-gated, voltage-gated and other ion channels; carrier proteins; drug-receptor activity; drug-enzyme interaction; therapeutic index
2 Using named examples, differentiate between the actions of agonistic and antagonistic drugs
3 Discuss the relationship between a drug's minimum effective concentration, toxic concentration level and therapeutic range
4 Differentiate between drug potency and drug efficacy
5 Using named examples, critically examine the factors which may affect the pharmacodynamic properties of drugs

---

## INTRODUCTION

The aim of this chapter is to explore the principles of pharmacodynamics. Pharmacodynamics is a branch of pharmacology. It is the study of the biochemical and physiological effects of drugs, the mechanisms of drug action and the relationship between drug concentration and effect.

## PRINCIPLES OF DRUG ACTION

A drug works to produce the desired effect by principally influencing normal physiological pathways or processes (see Table 6.1, which includes some pharmacodynamic actions).

**Table 6.1** Principles of drug action

| Drug action | Drug effect and examples |
| --- | --- |
| *Stimulation*: Selective enhancement of the level of activity of specialised cells so that a physiological pathway or system is stimulated | Pilocarpine stimulates salivary glands<br>Adrenaline and heart |
| *Inhibition/depression*: The activity of a physiological pathway or system is depressed or inhibited | Barbiturates depress CNS – e.g. thiopentone, phenobarbitone<br>Anxiolytics – e.g. diazepam |
| *Replacement*: Use of natural metabolites, hormones or other substances for deficiency states, which results in disease | Levodopa in Parkinsonism<br>Iron in anaemia |
| *Cytotoxic*: Cell death for invading microbes – e.g. bacteria, virus, fungal infections or neoplasms | Antibacterials – e.g. penicillin; antivirals – e.g. zidovudine in the treatment of human immunodeficiency virus; chemotherapy drugs – e.g. cancer treatment |
| *Modulation*: A group of drugs which bind to cell receptors to change their form and therefore the normal and anticipated response to the biological substances | Benzodiazepines – e.g. diazepam – which modulate GABA-A receptors in the brain |

In the prescribing of drugs for the prevention or management of disease and related signs and symptoms, principal drug actions should outweigh the side effects or risk of adverse reactions.

## SIDE EFFECTS AND ADVERSE DRUG RESPONSES

As well as producing desired effects, the action of the drug may result in known side effects.

The World Health Organization (WHO) defines a side effect as 'any unintended effect of a pharmaceutical product occurring at doses normally used by a patient which is related to the pharmacological properties of the drug' (World Health Organization, 2002). If we refer to the BNF, side effects are detailed as common or very common or uncommon and are generally anticipated as a potential, known consequence of the drug.

To offer an example, side effects for the opioid group of drugs are cited in the BNF as:

*Common or very common*: Arrhythmias; confusion; constipation; dizziness; drowsiness; dry mouth; euphoric mood; flushing; hallucination; headache; hyperhidrosis; miosis; nausea (more common on initiation); palpitations; respiratory depression (with high doses); skin reactions; urinary retention; vertigo; vomiting (more common on initiation); withdrawal syndrome

*Uncommon*: Drug dependence; dysphoria

Side effects are generally a consequence of the drug acting on the human body in additional ways to those intended for the site of action.

Take propranolol, for example, which is commonly known as a beta-blocker to reduce blood pressure. It acts as a nonselective, competitive antagonist at beta-adrenergic receptors, binding with high affinity to both beta-1 and beta-2 receptor subtypes. Beta-1 adrenergic receptors are located on cardiac muscle cells. Propranolol therefore acts to reduce the effect of adrenaline-binding on cardiac cells to reduce heart rate and blood pressure. However, propranolol also blocks beta-2 receptors in the bronchioles, which causes bronchoconstriction as a known side effect and is therefore contraindicated in asthma.

Another example is morphine sulphate, an opioid analgesic which exerts its pharmacological effect as an agonist at mu (μ) receptors principally found in the central nervous system. However, whilst the pain pathway is interrupted and pain is managed, morphine sulphate also binds to mu receptors in the gastrointestinal walls to reduce motility of the gut, leading to constipation. Also, morphine sulphate affects the respiratory centres in the pons varolii and medulla oblongata in the brainstem leading to respiratory depression.

The occurrence of side effects is variable and unpredictable. On occasions, side effects may be delayed with the long-term use of a drug or occur because of drug–drug and drug–food interactions as discussed in Chapter 4. Side effects can also be due to intentional or non-intentional overdose, medication errors, abuse, misuse or drug withdrawal. The words misuse and abuse have been used here, and it is useful to consider their distinctions. Whilst misuse is often an umbrella term used in clinical practice because it is less judgemental, it generally refers to the incorrect use of medicines without the intention to cause harm, such as taking an incorrect dose or sharing prescriptions. In contrast, abuse involves the intentional use of a medicine for non-therapeutic purposes, often to achieve a desired psychoactive effect, and is more commonly associated with addiction and dependency.

Several definitions of an 'adverse drug reaction' are published with definitions debated at length. The Medicines and Healthcare products Regulatory Agency (MHRA, 2024) define an adverse drug reaction as 'an unwanted side effect' caused by 'any medicine, vaccine, herbal or complementary remedy'. Under the new EU Directive 2010/84/EU1 that came into force in July 2012, the term 'adverse drug reaction' (ADR) is defined as:

> a response to a medicinal product that is noxious and unintended effects resulting not only from the authorised use of a medicinal product at normal doses, but also from medication errors and uses outside the terms of the marketing authorisation, including the misuse, off-label use and abuse of the medicinal product.
>
> (European Parliament and Council of the European Union, 2010)

An ADR is a response to a medicinal product which is noxious and unintended. Response in this context means that a causal relationship between a medicinal product and an adverse event is at least a reasonable possibility.

Adverse reactions may arise from use of the product within or outside the terms of the marketing authorisation or from occupational exposure. Conditions of use outside the marketing authorisation include off-label use, overdose, misuse, abuse and medication errors. The reaction may be a known side effect of the drug, or it may be new and previously unrecognised.

ADRs are also reported as:

- Augmented pharmacological effects
- Bizarre, unpredictable and uncommon
- Chronic effects seen in prolonged drug use
- Delayed effects
- End of treatment effects seen once the drug has been stopped (adverse withdrawal effects)

The occurrence of an adverse drug reaction warrants action whether that is withdrawal of the drug or alteration of the dosage regimen. Reporting of ADRs to the MHRA through the Yellow Card reporting system allows for the national collation of data and in extreme cases withdrawal of the drug's marketing authorisation.

### PAUSE AND REFLECT 6.1

Examine the concept of adverse drug reactions (ADRs). Choose a medication and research its most common and serious ADRs. How are ADRs reported and monitored in clinical practice to ensure patient safety?

## THE PRINCIPLES OF DRUG ACTION

The following section explores pharmacodynamics (i.e. the principal modes of action of drugs) and provides examples.

### Cell Receptors

The plasma membrane of a human cell is selectively permeable, which helps control what moves in and out of the cell (see Figure 6.1). As explained in Chapter 1, the cell membrane is a bilayer of phospholipids, studded with proteins. These proteins perform a variety of different functions and are defined as 'receptors'.

Receptors specifically recognise and bind to ligands. A ligand is a molecule that binds to a receptor to produce a biological response. Ligands can be drugs, hormones or neurotransmitters.

# PRINCIPLES OF PHARMACODYNAMICS

There is a wide range of receptors, which share essential functions:

- To recognise and bind to the body's own chemical messengers, such as hormones and neurotransmitters
- To convert the binding process into a signal that the cell will respond to in some way

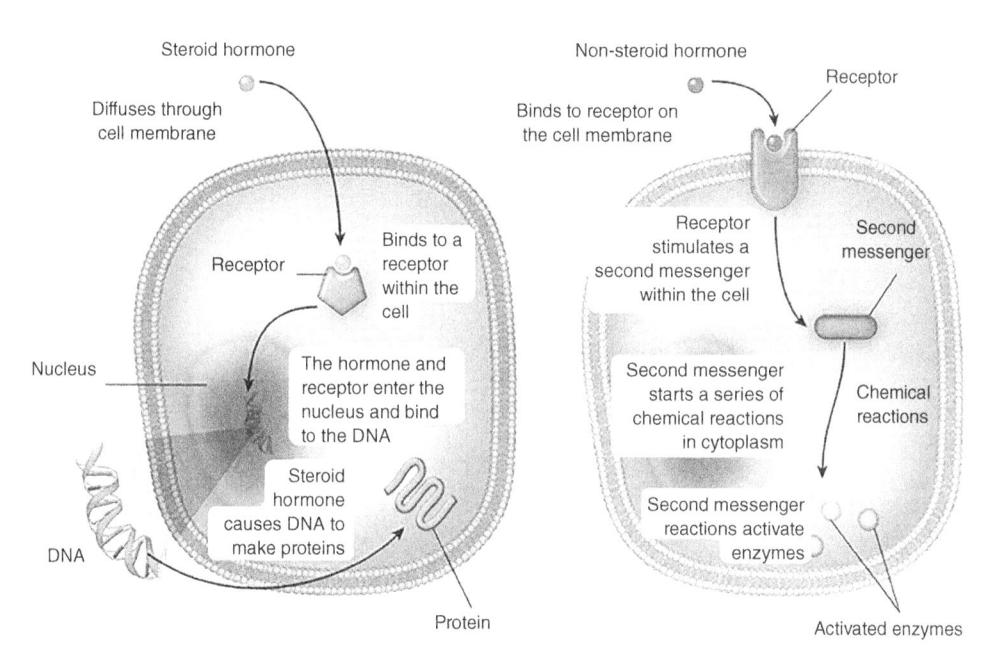

**Figure 6.1** Cell receptors

**Table 6.2** Range of receptors

| Receptor type | Description | Examples |
| --- | --- | --- |
| Channel-linked receptors or ligand-gated ion channels | Proteins located in the cell membrane that contain a pore or channel and regulate the flow of selected ions (namely Na+, K+, Ca2+, and Cl- across the plasma membrane. These channels are known as 'ligand-gated' because they are activated by a chemical or ligand binding to them which results in opening or closing of the channel (in contrast to 'voltage-gated' channels that respond to changes in membrane potential) | Nicotine acetylcholine receptors Gamma-aminobutyric acid (GABA) receptors selectively conduct Cl- through their pores or channels, which plays a part in neuronal inhibition in the amygdala, leading to fewer excitatory signals to other areas of the brain, providing a reduction in the physiological and psychological markers of stress and anxiety. Benzodiazepines (e.g. diazepam) enhance the binding of GABA to its receptor activating the Cl- channel, allowing for the neuronal inhibition which reduces anxiety. An example of voltage gated ion channels is the Na+ channel. These are responsible for the creation of action potentials of long duration, and therefore are targets of local anaesthetics, such as lidocaine |

*(Continued)*

**Table 6.2** (Continued)

| Receptor type | Description | Examples |
| --- | --- | --- |
| G protein-coupled receptors | The largest class of cell membrane-bound receptors. They respond to a wide variety of extracellular signals, for example hormones or neurotransmitters. This initiates intracellular signalling cascade through secondary messengers to regulate many physiological functions | Muscarinic acetylcholine receptors Beta-adrenoreceptors Dopamine receptors 5-hydroxytryptamine (serotonin) receptors Opioid receptors |
| Enzyme-linked receptors | A transmembrane receptor where the binding of an extracellular ligand causes enzymatic activity on the intracellular side | Insulin receptors |
| Intracellular steroid or nuclear hormone receptors | Intracellular and known as 'nuclear receptors'. Binding of a ligand promotes or inhibits synthesis of new proteins, which may take hours or days to promote a biological effect | Steroid hormone receptors Thyroid hormone receptors Vitamin D receptors |

However, in the unbound state, a receptor is functionally 'silent'. The range of receptors can be divided into four groups (see Table 6.2).

To explain the action of receptors and ligand interactions, synaptic transmission between neurones in the brain will be explained as an example. Figure 6.2 illustrates the physical properties at the end of one axon fibre and its connection with another. The gap between the two neurones is called the 'synaptic cleft'.

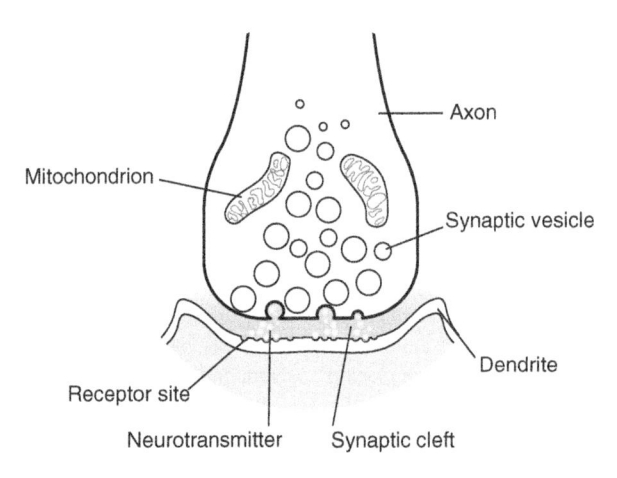

**Figure 6.2** Synaptic transmission

When the nerve impulse arrives at the terminal end of the first neurone (i.e. the 'synaptic bulb'), synaptic vesicles which contain the neurotransmitter (the naturally occurring ligand or endogenous substance) moves down to the pre-synaptic membrane. Through a process of exocytosis, the neurotransmitter is released into the synaptic cleft and then binds to its respective receptor on the post-synaptic membrane, forming a ligand-receptor complex rather like a lock and key system. The three-dimensional shape of the ligand molecule acts like the key and must be an exact fit for the target/receptor (the lock) to activate it. Therefore, the interactions between the ligand and its target (i.e. the receptor) are highly specific and based on physical shape interaction.

The ligand–receptor binding activates a cellular response (i.e. the key opens the door), in this case neurotransmission. It may be that there is a conformational change in the physical properties of the cell membrane (e.g. the opening of voltage-gated channels or a chain response within the cell). Once neurotransmission has taken place, the ligand is either destroyed by enzymes or reabsorbed into the synaptic bulb (uptake) by binding to pre-synaptic receptors. The neurotransmitter is then repackaged for future use.

Drugs are developed to modulate and influence activity at receptor sites and therefore alter the extent to which neurotransmission takes place. This is achieved in the following ways:

1. Increasing the level of ligand (endogenous substance) by administering a drug which is the ligand or is pharmaceutically developed to mimic the chemical structure of the ligand molecule
2. Increasing the re-uptake of the ligand through the pre-synaptic receptors to reduce the amount of ligand present in the synaptic cleft and therefore reduce receptor activation
3. Decreasing the re-uptake of the ligand through the pre-synaptic receptors to increase the amount of ligand present in the synaptic cleft and therefore increase receptor activation
4. Blocking the post-synaptic receptors to reduce ligand–receptor activation

Interactions between drugs and receptors can occur in a variety of ways and are classified as *agonistic, antagonistic* or *allosteric modulated*.

## An Agonist

An agonist is a drug that binds to a receptor and activates it, producing a biological response. An agonist drug therefore mimics the naturally occurring ligand or endogenous substance. If we return to our example of synaptic transmission, an agonist drug would bind to a dopamine receptor in the same way as dopamine does and activate the same cellular response. To offer an example: Parkinson's disease is a result of a lack of dopamine in the centres of the brain which control movement. Symptoms of dopamine depletion include bradykinesia (slowing of movement), a resting tremor, muscle rigidity and impaired balance and coordination. Dopamine agonists include apomorphine, ropinirole and pramipexole, which bind to the post-synaptic dopamine receptors and increase neurotransmission.

## A Full Agonist

A full agonist is a drug which can produce a maximum response that the target system or tissue is capable of. A full agonist effect does not necessarily need to occur when all receptors are occupied. A full agonist effect can happen at different doses with only a fraction of the receptors occupied. Figure 6.3 illustrates this, demonstrating several full agonists with different potencies.

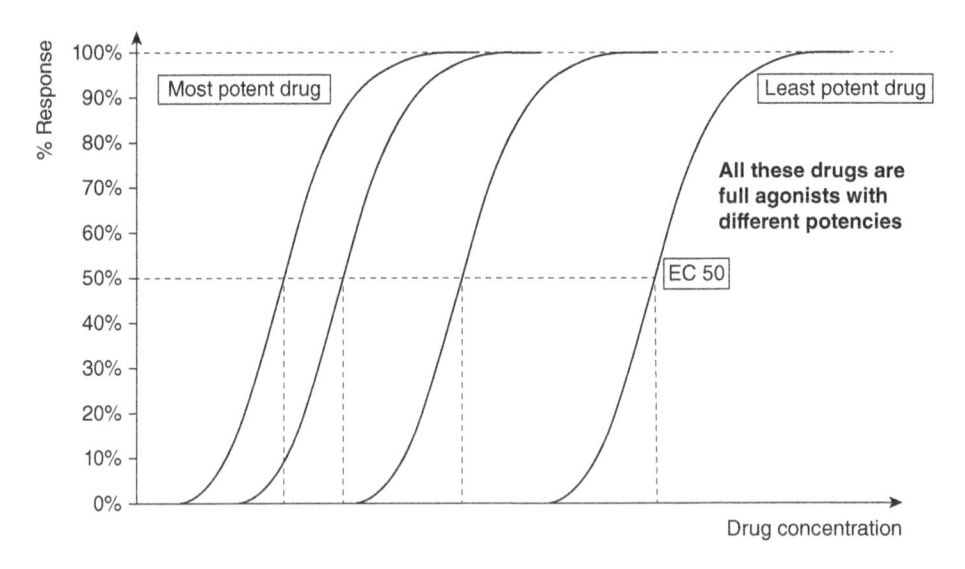

**Figure 6.3** Full agonists with different potencies

**Potency** refers to the concentration, amount or strength of a drug that is required to have an effect. A highly potent drug will require a lower dose than a less potent drug as shown in Figure 6.3. Alprazolam and diazepam are both benzodiazepines and are used in the treatment of anxiety. However, alprazolam is more potent and therefore an individual will need a smaller dose of alprazolam than diazepam to produce a response. In fact, it is thought that 0.5 mg of alprazolam is approximately equivalent to 5 mg diazepam.

## A Partial Agonist

Partial agonists are drugs that bind to a receptor but, compared to a full agonist, do not have full efficacy at that receptor. **Efficacy** refers to the ability of a drug to activate a response once bound to a receptor. A drug with a higher efficacy will produce a bigger effect on a cell than a drug with lower efficacy even if both drugs have bound to the same number of receptors on the cell. A partial agonist has a lower efficacy than a full agonist and therefore produces a lesser response. For example, tramadol is a partial agonist at opioid receptors. It has lower efficacy than morphine in the management of severe pain, but an advantage is that it also has a lesser effect in its capacity to cause respiratory depression.

Partial agonists, when binding at the receptor, may also block it from being bound by a full agonist and can therefore act as a partial (competitive) antagonist to that receptor.

## An Inverse Agonist

An inverse agonist binds to a receptor and causes a decrease in signalling at the receptor and produces effects that are opposite to those of an agonist. Only a few types of receptors in the body have been the subject of research and have identified ligands that act as inverse agonists. This means that there are very few, if any, drugs that act as inverse agonists as their primary desired pharmacological effect and that are in true medical use.

One example in use is diphenhydramine, which is an older $H_1$-antihistamine. $H_1$-antihistamines are not structurally like histamine and so do not block histamine from binding to its receptor. Instead, they attach to different sites on the receptor, producing effects opposite to those of histamine. Therefore, $H_1$-antihistamines are considered inverse agonists because they elicit the opposite response on the receptor compared to histamine. In sources they are often named histamine antagonists, but it may be more correct to refer to them as histamine antagonists and it should be noted that drugs like diphenhydramine have actions at a few other receptor targets as well.

Some drugs, such as naloxone, which is known as an opioid antagonist, can also act as an inverse agonist under specific binding circumstances when an agonist opioid is present. For most clinical purposes, it is sufficient to focus on naloxone's role as an antagonist. However, its ability to act as an inverse agonist may (and only may) enhance its effectiveness in overdose cases by mitigating certain withdrawal effects, such as withdrawal jumping. Withdrawal jumping specifically refers to a characteristic behaviour where individuals experiencing opioid withdrawal exhibit repetitive, involuntary leg movements, often described as 'jumping' or 'kicking'. In clinical settings, observing withdrawal jumping can be a sign that a patient is experiencing severe opioid withdrawal and may require medical intervention to manage their symptoms effectively.

In terms of true inverse agonists an example would be Ro15-4513. This drug, known as a '$\beta$-carboline' compound, is a class of psychoactive alkaloid. It is classified as a partial inverse agonist at the benzodiazepine binding site of GABA-A receptors. This means that it can produce effects opposite to those of benzodiazepines, such as increased anxiety and convulsions, while also blocking some of the effects of benzodiazepines. Whilst this might seem as if it could be used to treat overdose, it is better to use an antagonist with a higher infinity for GABA receptors than agonist benzodiazepines. This is because of the difficulty of using inverse agonists. For example, in this situation,

Ro15-4513 could have such an inverse agonism that the GABA receptor could no longer support brain homeostasis and cause severe seizures or profound anxiety that would be very difficult to treat.

## An Antagonist

An antagonist is a drug that binds to a receptor but does not activate it. It stops or blocks the biological response and may be *competitive* (reversible) or *non-competitive* (irreversible). An antagonist will effectively 'sit' in the receptor site, occupy the receptor, so that the naturally occurring ligand or endogenous substance or agonist drug cannot activate the receptor. No cellular response is seen.

Returning to the lock and key hypothesis, the key fits the lock but does not activate it (i.e. the door does not open).

Competitive (reversible) antagonism is the most common. Here a drug competes with an agonist for its binding site, limiting the amount of agonist that can bind to the receptor at the same time.

To return to our example of dopamine as a neurotransmitter. Whilst there are many hypotheses as to the complex aetiology of schizophrenia, dopamine hyperactivity in specific areas of the brain is thought be a contributing factor in the presentation of the clinical manifestations. The second-generation anti-psychotics (atypical) – olanzapine, quetiapine and risperidone – are examples of dopamine antagonists, which act as reversible, competitive 'blockers' at dopamine receptors. This reduces dopamine–dopamine receptor binding and ultimately dopamine hyperactivity at the synapse.

Another example is naloxone, which is administered to reverse respiratory depression, sedation and other side effects of opioid overdose. Naloxone is *a reversible, competitive antagonist*. It attaches to opioid receptor sites which in turn blocks the binding of opioids (e.g. morphine and diamorphine (heroin)). However, it is important to understand that competitive or reversible antagonists frequently bind to, and unbind from, the receptor, allowing the agonist to replace the antagonist whilst in the unbound state. This allows the antagonist's effects to be overcome by the addition of more agonist.

Another example of a receptor antagonist is the SSRI group of drugs (e.g. citalopram, fluoxetine and paroxetine) prescribed for their antidepressant action. The SSRIs 'block' the pre-synaptic membrane receptors so that serotonin is not reabsorbed back into the synaptic bulb. The result is that more serotonin remains in the synaptic cleft for longer with a resultant increase serotonin-receptor binding in parts of the brain that control mood.

The group of drugs collectively called beta-blockers (e.g. atenolol, bisoprolol and propranolol) indicated in the control of hypertension are competitive antagonists at the beta-adrenoreceptors in the heart. Adrenaline, a naturally occurring ligand produced in response to the activation of the sympathetic nervous system during flight and fight, binds to beta-adrenoreceptors which increases heart rate and cardiac output with a resultant increase in blood pressure. This means that less adrenaline–adrenoreceptor binding can occur, which will ultimately reduce blood pressure.

Curare, a neurotoxin, is a non-depolarising neuromuscular blocking agent (NMBA). At the neuromuscular junction (i.e. the junction between a neuron and a muscle cell), acetylcholine is released into the synaptic cleft to facilitate communication from the synaptic bulb at the preganglionic neurone and binds to nicotinic receptors on the post-synaptic membrane. This results in depolarisation and muscular contraction. However, when curare is present, it competes for the nicotinic receptor sites and 'blocks' the binding of acetylcholine, leading to muscular paralysis (see Figure 6.4). This principle is adopted in clinical practice when muscle paralysis is required during surgery or to support ventilatory support. Atracurium and vecuronium are non-depolarising muscular blocking agents administered intravenously, which competitively bind to cholinergic receptor sites.

Atropine binds reversibly to the muscarinic receptors found in postganglionic, parasympathetic neurones. It is therefore defined as an 'antimuscarinic agent' by competitively blocking the acetylcholine receptors in smooth muscle and cardiac muscle (see Figure 6.4). Because activation of the parasympathetic division of the autonomic nervous system by acetylcholine-muscarinic receptor binding normally results in the lowering of the heart rate, the effect of atropine effectively reverses this to cause an increase in sinoatrial activity and cardiac conduction to increase the heart rate.

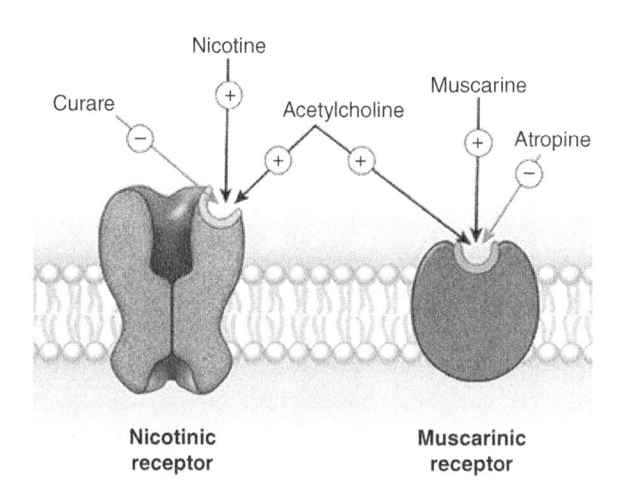

**Figure 6.4** Nicotinic and muscarinic receptors

Non-competitive antagonists (irreversible) also bind to the same site as an agonist but unbind very slowly or not at all. They therefore reduce the action of an agonist, regardless of how much agonist is present. One example of a non-competitive antagonist (irreversible) is phenoxybenzamine. Phenoxybenzamine is a medication used primarily to treat conditions like pheochromocytoma (a tumour of the adrenal gland) and hypertension associated with certain conditions like neuroblastoma. Phenoxybenzamine irreversibly binds to and blocks alpha-adrenergic receptors. These receptors are normally activated by adrenaline and noradrenaline which are neurotransmitters that play a role in the 'fight or flight' response of the sympathetic nervous system. By irreversibly blocking alpha-adrenergic receptors, phenoxybenzamine reduces the action of adrenaline and noradrenaline, leading to vasodilation (relaxation of blood vessels) and ultimately lowering blood pressure. Because phenoxybenzamine binds irreversibly to its target receptors, its effects cannot be easily reversed once the drug has been administered. This irreversibility is a characteristic feature of non-competitive antagonists.

## In Summary

Table 6.3 summarises the definitions of an agonist and antagonist drug, with Figure 6.5 illustrating principles of action at the receptor site.

**Table 6.3** Agonist vs antagonist

| | |
|---|---|
| AGONIST | A drug which mimics the naturally occurring ligand, forms a ligand-receptor complex and activates a cellular response |
| ANTAGONIST | A drug which binds to the receptor, does not 'fit' exactly but 'blocks' the naturally occurring ligand from binding. Cellular response is not activated |

*Source*: Wikimedia Commons

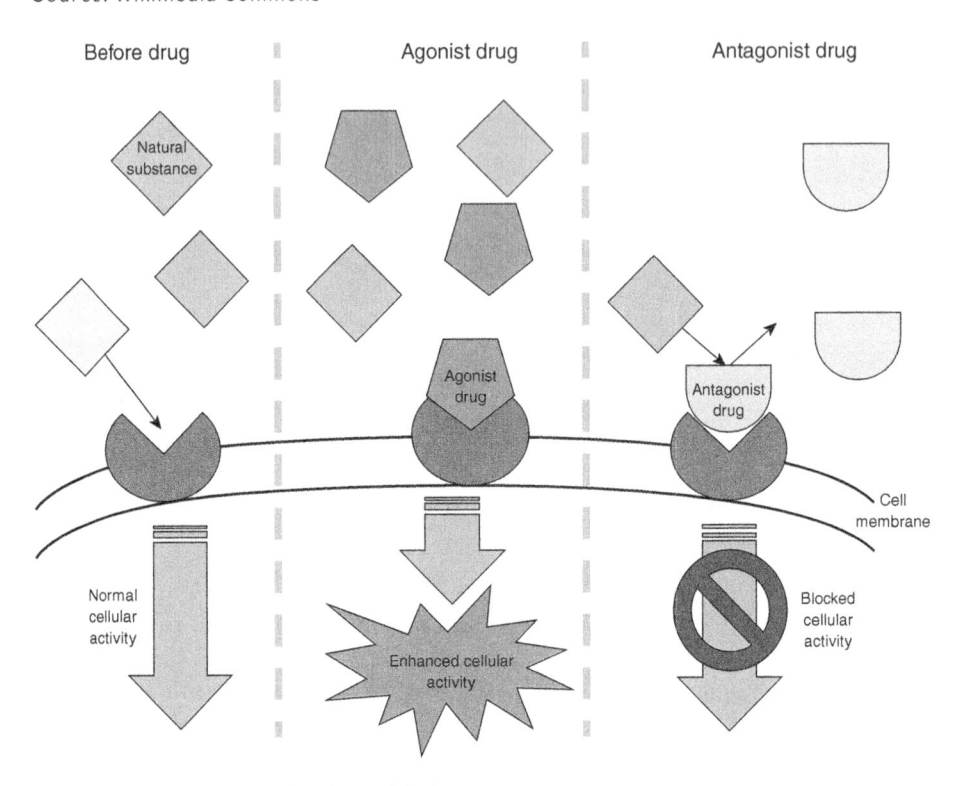

**Figure 6.5** Agonist and antagonist drugs

*Source*: Wikipedia under a Creative Commons Attribution-Share Alike 3.0 license

## An Allosteric Modulator

These are drugs that bind to a site on the receptor different from where the agonist binds but still influence the action of that receptor. They can activate the receptor on their own or they may increase or decrease the likelihood of an agonist binding to a receptor, enhancing or reducing the effects when it does bind. They can therefore affect the **affinity** of a drug. Affinity refers to the property of a drug or ligand in its ability to bind to a receptor. A drug's affinity is constant and unique for the drug–receptor binding. Drugs or endogenous (natural) substances need to bind long and tightly enough to initiate and facilitate the cellular response. Substances that bind very tightly to their receptors are described as having a high affinity. Drugs with a high affinity will bind first over other drugs or the endogenous substance. This property of affinity is very important and can be utilised by pharmacologists, particularly when the natural endogenous substance is in abundance and is the cause of the problem or symptoms the individual experiences. For example, naloxone has a high affinity for opioid receptors in the central nervous system, particularly the mu–opioid receptors. When administered, naloxone competes with opioids to bind to these receptors. Due to its higher affinity, naloxone effectively displaces opioids from the receptor sites, reversing their effects. By blocking the action of opioids at the receptor level, naloxone rapidly reverses the respiratory depression, sedation and other central nervous system effects caused by opioid overdose, potentially saving the individual's life. The high affinity of naloxone for opioid receptors allows it to effectively outcompete opioids for receptor binding, making it a crucial intervention in opioid overdose situations.

Drugs that have very high affinity and are poorly reversible following binding to the receptor often behave as antagonists, preventing the ability of the naturally occurring signalling molecule from activating the receptor. There is another drug that is useful in overdose situations that is a good example of this: flumazenil is a benzodiazepine receptor antagonist used to reverse the effects of benzodiazepine overdose or to rapidly reverse the sedative effects of benzodiazepines during medical procedures. It has a very high affinity for the benzodiazepine binding site on the GABA-A receptor. When administered, flumazenil competes with benzodiazepines for binding to the benzodiazepine site on the GABA-A receptor. Due to its high affinity and poor reversibility, flumazenil effectively displaces benzodiazepines from the receptor sites, blocking their action. By antagonising the effects of benzodiazepines at the receptor level, flumazenil rapidly reverses sedation and other central nervous system depressant effects caused by benzodiazepine overdose or excessive use. The high affinity and poor reversibility of flumazenil binding to the benzodiazepine receptor make it an effective antagonist in reversing the effects of benzodiazepines.

Another important property of any drug to consider is its **selectivity** and **specificity**. These terms are often used interchangeably but they do have distinct actions.

## Selectivity

Selectivity refers to a drug's strong preference for its intended target over all other targets.

Drugs vary in how selective they are for a particular receptor. Some are highly selective and activate a single receptor, whilst others may activate a wide variety of receptors in different body systems (see Table 6.4).

**Table 6.4** Selectivity of a drug

| Degree of selectivity | Example of drug | Action |
| --- | --- | --- |
| *Relatively nonselective drugs*, which may impact a range of different tissues or organs | Propranolol (beta blocker) | Block both beta1 and beta2 receptors and so affect the heart, lungs, vascular smooth muscles, kidneys, and gastro-intestinal tract |
| *Relatively selective drugs* | Non-steroidal anti-inflammatory drugs – e.g. aspirin or ibuprofen | Target any areas where inflammation is present |
| *Highly selective drugs*, which mainly affect a single organ or systems | Digoxin | Targets heart to improve its pumping efficiency |

The selectivity of a drug has significant clinical implications and can affect an individual's drug regimen. For example, isoprenaline a drug used to control asthma, is a non-selective $\beta$-adrenergic agonist and interacts with both $\beta_1$- and $\beta_2$-adrenergic receptors in the heart and smooth muscle tissues. Therefore it affects not only the bronchioles but also the cardiac muscles. This may be a concern if the patient has cardiac problems. In this case, salbutamol may be considered a more suitable drug as it is a selective $\beta_2$ adrenergic agonist. This means it will specifically target smooth muscle cells in the bronchioles leading to bronchodilation and relief of asthmatic symptoms.

## Specificity

Specificity describes the extent to which a drug produces *only* the desired therapeutic effect but does not cause any other physiological changes and therefore has minimal side effects. A drug with high specificity has a strong drug–receptor interaction. In comparison, drugs with low specificity have a weak drug–receptor interaction and thus may have unintended consequences.

For example, amiodarone, an anti-arrhythmic drug, demonstrates low specificity, affecting multiple ion channels and causing various side effects. On the other hand, omeprazole, a proton-pump inhibitor, shows high specificity by selectively inhibiting gastric acid secretion without impacting other physiological processes.

However, the unwanted side effects due to low specificity may lead to new and desired effects. A classic example of this is sildenafil (Viagra) which was originally developed to treat hypertension and angina. It was not particularly effective, but an observed side effect has become the new targeted role of the drug.

## Carrier Protons as Target Sites of Drug Action

In pharmacodynamics, which is the study of how medications exert their effects on the body, drugs that affect carrier proteins or pumps play an important role. Controlling the movement of ions, nutrients and medications, carrier proteins and pumps are essential components of cell membranes that transport various substances across the membrane in a way that would be against a diffusion gradient and could be achieved by simple facilitated diffusion. When drugs target these transport systems, they can affect the movement of substances into and out of cells, resulting in therapeutic effects.

These transport systems are specific to particular molecules or types of molecules found in the body involved in homeostasis or control. In numerous ways, drugs can interact with these transporters. For example, some drugs can inhibit the activity of specific carrier proteins or pumps. This can reduce the transmembrane transport of essential nutrients, ions and other substances. Proton pump inhibitors (PPIs), for instance, inhibit the proton pump responsible for gastric acid secretion, thereby reducing stomach acid production.

Another example of the drug inhibiting the pump is antidepressants. They affect the re-uptake of neurotransmitters, such as serotonin and norepinephrine (see Figure 6.6), by inhibiting transporters responsible for their removal from the synaptic cleft. This increases neurotransmitter availability and can improve mood regulation. Although it is important to note that the therapeutic action of antidepressants work is not solely due to the increase in neurotransmitters in the synapse, it is another good illustration of drugs which target pumps that move a molecule found in the body.

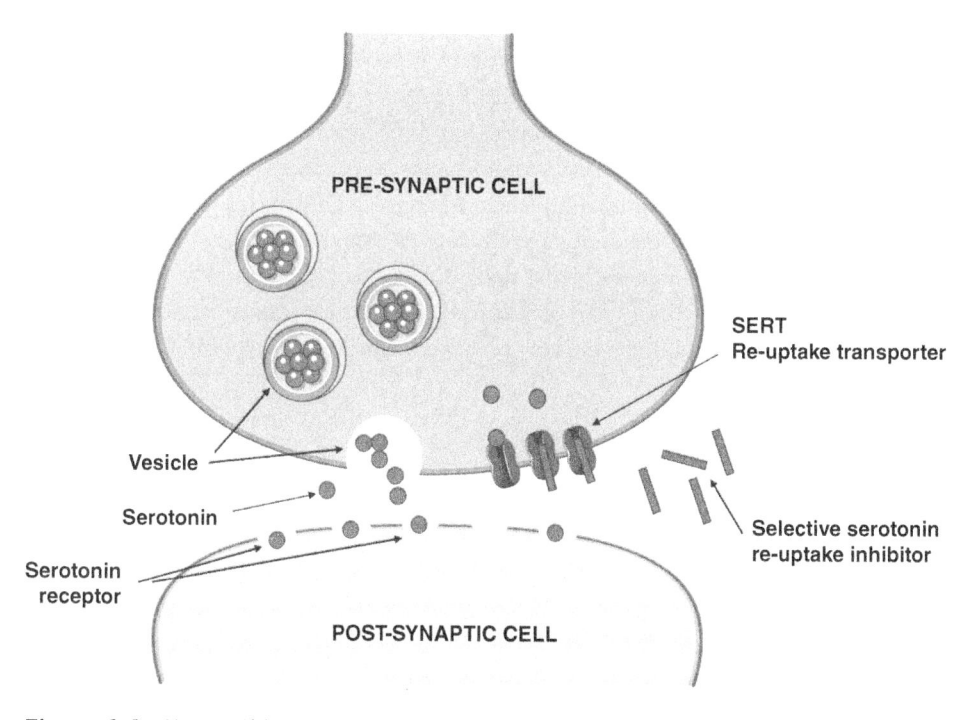

**Figure 6.6** How antidepressants inhibit the pump

*Source*: Created using Servier Medical Art. Servier Medical Art is licenced under a Creative Commons Attribution 3.0 Unported License https://creativecommons.org/licenses/by/3.0/.

Other substances may activate carrier proteins or pumps, thereby facilitating the transport of specific molecules. **Diuretics**, for example, can activate sodium–potassium transporters in the kidney tubules, resulting in increased sodium and water excretion via urine. This reduces fluid retention, making them useful for treating conditions like hypertension and oedema.

In most cases it is obvious that drugs such as antidepressants that increase serotonin levels might lead to serotonin syndrome due to high concentrations of serotonin resulting in agitation, confusion and restlessness, or in the case of diuretics electrolyte imbalances due to over-excretion of electrolytes affecting heart rhythm.

However, medications can have adverse effects at sites other than their primary target. The class of anti-cancer pharmaceuticals known as P-glycoprotein (P-gp) inhibitors is a notable example of a drug that interacts with transporters to induce cellular toxicity. P-gp is a transporter protein that actively pumps toxins and medications out of cells, thereby protecting cells from toxicity. Overexpression of P-gp in cancer cells can contribute to drug resistance by decreasing intracellular chemotherapeutic agent concentrations.

Verapamil is one well-known P-gp inhibitor. In addition to its primary use as a **calcium channel blocker** for the treatment of hypertension and cardiac arrhythmias, verapamil inhibits P-gp. This might be seen to be beneficial as this P-gp inhibition can increase chemotherapy drug concentrations within cancer cells, but it can also increase chemotherapy drug exposure in normal tissues, which may increase the adverse drug reactions associated with chemotherapy treatments. Examples of chemotherapy drugs that interact with verapamil are doxorubicin, vinblastine and paclitaxel.

Whilst currently in this example the concern is about toxic drug interactions, verapamil has been investigated as an adjuvant therapy to improve the efficacy of certain anti-cancer drugs in the treatment of cancer.

Verapamil can be used alongside these same anti-cancer drugs (doxorubicin, vinblastine, and paclitaxel) in combination chemotherapy regimens for the treatment of specific forms of cancer. These drugs are substrates of P-gp and are actively pumped out of cancer cells by this transporter, potentially diminishing their efficacy. By inhibiting P-gp with verapamil, intracellular concentrations of these drugs can be increased, resulting in enhanced cytotoxic effects on cancer cells and the potential to overcome drug resistance.

---

## PAUSE AND REFLECT 6.2

Combination therapy using two or more drugs together is a strategy used throughout pharmacotherapeutics, not just in chemotherapy. Examine the use of combination therapy in treating diseases. Choose a condition (we suggest pain, antimicrobials or hypertension) that is commonly treated with multiple drugs and explain the rationale behind using combination therapy. How does this approach improve treatment outcomes?

The use of P-gp inhibitors in the treatment of cancer is the subject of ongoing research and clinical investigation, as the trade-off between increased drug efficacy and toxicity must be carefully managed. This example demonstrates how drug interactions with transporters can influence drug distribution and cellular responses, both in terms of therapeutic effects and potential toxicity.

## Enzyme Inhibition as a Target Site of Drug Action

Many physiological systems employ enzymes as biological catalysts. Drugs have been developed to influence the rate and extent of these enzyme-catalysed reactions. A drug which is termed an 'enzyme inhibitor' will affect enzyme-induced reactions in the body. The drug, the 'enzyme inhibitor', will compete for the 'active site' of the enzyme and therefore block the enzyme from acting on the substrate. In this way, the normal enzyme-catalysed reaction cannot occur (see Figure 6.7).

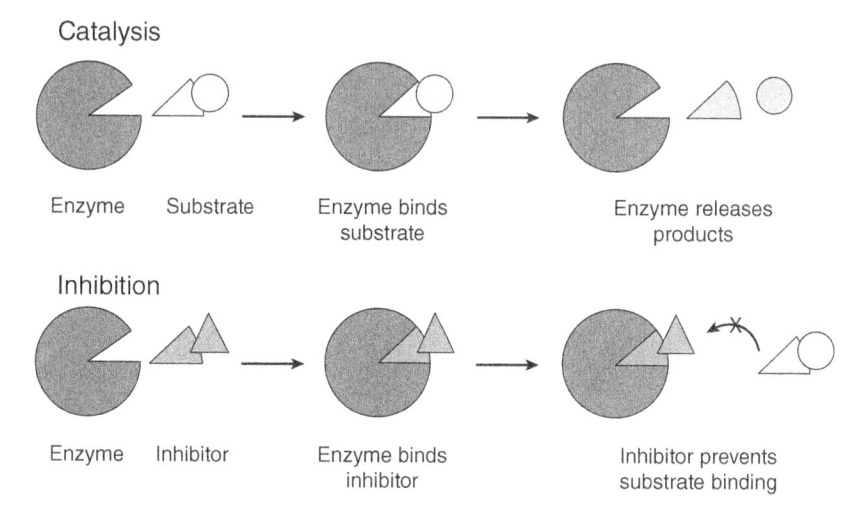

**Figure 6.7** Enzyme catalysis vs enzyme inhibitor
*Source*: Wikipedia under a Creative Commons Attribution-Share Alike 4.0 license.

We now explore some examples of drugs which act as enzyme inhibitors.

### ACE Inhibitors Such as Captopril, Enalapril, Lisinopril

In the maintenance of blood pressure, the production of renin from the juxtaglomerular cells of the kidney stimulates the conversion of angiotensinogen (produced in the liver) to angiotensin I. Angiotensin I is converted to angiotensin II by the angiotensin-converting enzyme (ACE). Angiotensin II has several physiological functions which include the stimulation of production of aldosterone from the adrenal cortex. This acts on the nephron to increase sodium reabsorption, which increases water absorption and blood pressure. Angiotensin II also elevates blood pressure by causing peripheral vasoconstriction and increasing venous return to the heart.

The 'ACE inhibitor' group of drugs act by competitively inhibiting ACE by binding to its active site, so that angiotensin I is not converted to angiotensin II. The production of angiotensin II is therefore reduced, which means blood pressure is lowered.

## Aspirin and Inhibition of Cyclo-Oxygenase (COX-1 and COX-2)

When tissue damage occurs, there is a release of inflammatory mediators or chemicals (e.g. prostaglandins, bradykinins, histamine) which activate the nociceptors (pain receptors). The production of prostaglandin arises from the enzyme-catalysed reaction whereby COX-1 (cyclo-oxygenase I) and COX-2 converts arachidonic acid to prostaglandins and thromboxane, the latter involved in the clotting cascade (see Figure 6.8). The non-steroidal anti-inflammatory (NSAIDs) group of drugs (e.g. aspirin, ibuprofen) are COX-1 and COX-2 enzyme inhibitors. They act by blocking the conversion of arachidonic acid to prostaglandins and thromboxane. They are therefore indicated for pain and in preventing the aggregation of platelets (which in turn reduces the size of thrombus formation and risk of cardiovascular and cerebrovascular disease). However, prostaglandins have other functions elsewhere in the body. For example, prostaglandins support the production of mucus in the stomach to protect the gastric lining and have a protective function in the kidneys. This leads to the known side effect of gastric irritation or ulcer formation, or renal problems in the event of drug toxicity.

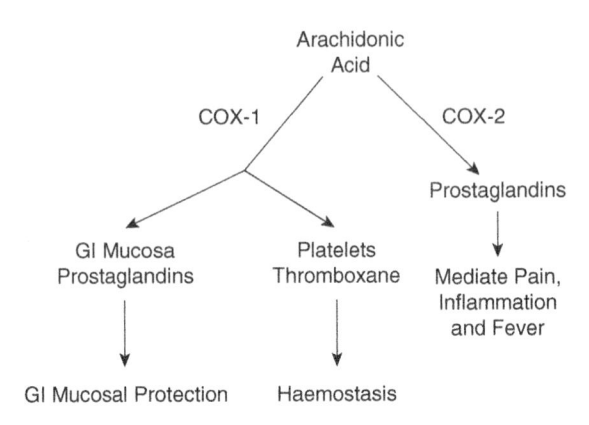

**Figure 6.8** Arachidonic acid metabolism pathways

The newer group of drugs termed COX-2 selective drugs (e.g. celecoxib or valdecoxib) only inhibit the action of COX-2 enzyme and therefore the gastrointestinal and renal side effects are not seen. They do, however, reduce the signs of inflammation and the associated pain experience.

## Monoamine Oxidase Inhibitors such as Selegiline, Isocarboxazid, Phenelzine

The monoamine oxidase (MAO) enzyme is responsible for the breakdown of the amine group of neurotransmitters in the brain (e.g. the catecholamines: dopamine, norepinephrine (noradrenaline) and epinephrine (adrenaline), and histamine and serotonin).

In depression, it is believed that there is a lack of noradrenaline or serotonin, and therefore if the breakdown of these neurotransmitters can be reduced, more remain in the synaptic cleft and neurotransmission can occur in the brain circuits which control mood. However, there are known dietary restrictions which include tyramine-containing foods (e.g. cured or salt dried meats, fermented soy products and aged cheeses). It is believed that tyramine displaces noradrenaline, adrenaline and dopamine from the pre-synaptic storage vesicles. This in turn elevates these levels in the body resulting in a hypertensive crisis and an increase in the heart rate.

### Anticholinesterases such as Neostigmine Bromide and Pyridostigmine Bromide

Anticholinesterases are commonly used in the treatment of myasthenia gravis. Myasthenia gravis is a chronic, autoimmune, neuromuscular condition which causes weakness of the voluntary muscles. During synaptic transmission at the neuromuscular junction, acetylcholine binds to acetylcholine receptors (cholinergic receptors) on the muscle cells resulting in muscular contraction. Once this has happened, the enzyme cholinesterase floods the synaptic cleft to metabolise acetylcholine. In myasthenia gravis, the thymus gland produces antibodies which bind to the cholinergic receptors on the muscle cells so that neuromuscular transmission cannot happen. The anticholinesterase group of drugs inhibit the action of the enzyme cholinesterase, which results in more acetylcholine remaining in the synaptic cleft. This facilitates neuromuscular transmission and contraction of voluntary muscles, reducing muscle weakness.

## CYTOTOXIC DRUG ACTION

A drug named as a 'cytotoxic' agent reflects its action as 'cell killing,' whether it targets an antigen that invades the body (e.g., bacteria or viruses) or neoplastic cells, such as those involved in tumour growth. However, one of the many challenges is that cytotoxic drugs need to directly kill the cell whilst at the same time safeguarding the human host cell.

In the treatment of microbial infection, drugs do this by specifically harnessing the unique physical and biochemical properties of the microbes in their action. Unfortunately, this does not mean that normal bacterial flora in the gut, for example, can be preserved.

### Antibacterial Drugs

A bacterium is a microbe that, as an antigen, can cause disease. There are several classifications of bacterial cells which have a unique, defining structure and function. Examples include alpha-haemolytic streptococci, *Bordatella pertussis* (whooping cough), *Neisseria meningitis* (meningococcus), *Mycobacterium tuberculosis*, *Clostridium botulinum* and *Clostridium difficile*. Whilst the shape, size and physical properties of bacteria will vary depending on the species, there are fundamental structures unique to bacteria (see Figure 6.9).

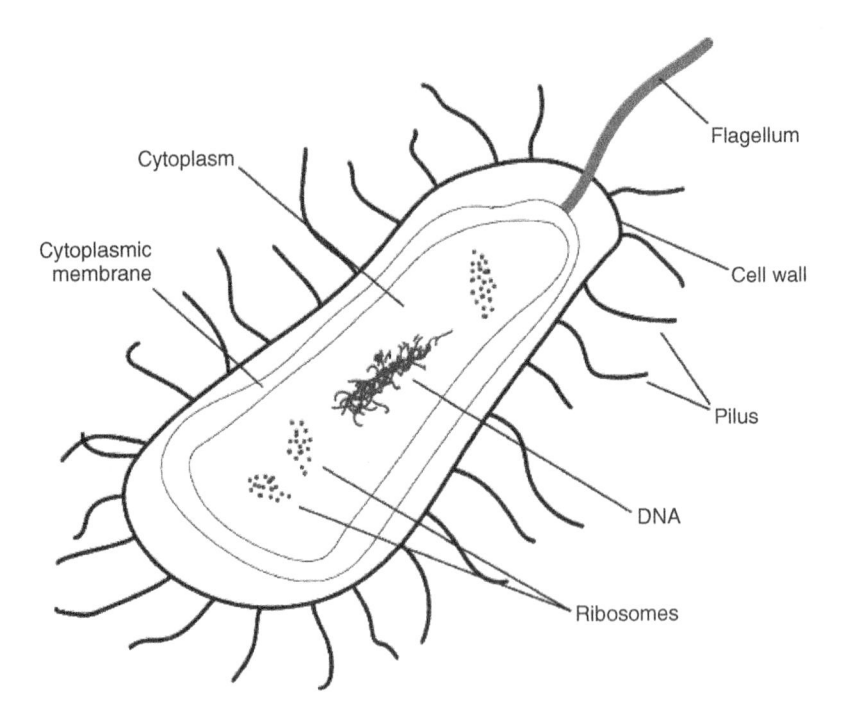

**Figure 6.9** A bacterium

Antibacterial drugs act through several mechanisms which harness these physical structures and properties to either halt the bacterial replication (bacteriostatic) or directly kill the bacteria (bactericidal). For example, bactericidal drugs (e.g. the beta-lactam antibiotics: penicillin derivatives, cephalosporins and vancomycin) affect the development of the bacterial cell wall or inhibit protein synthesis or folic acid (folate) production during bacterial reproduction or bacterial growth.

Bacteriostatic drugs (e.g. chloramphenicol) will halt bacterial growth by affecting DNA replication which in turn prevents bacterial growth or replication. The immune system can then more effectively eliminate the causative organism.

## Antiviral Drugs

A virus replicates within a host cell of the human. For example, hepatitis A replicates within the hepatocytes of the liver and the human immunodeficiency virus (HIV) in the helper-T lymphocyte, a white blood cell.

The replication cycle begins when the virus enters the specific human cell and effectively adopts this as its 'replication factory'. The steps include:

1 Attachment
2 Entry
3 Replication
4 Assembly
5 Release

Figure 6.10 shows how the virus enters the host cell by first attaching to a cell surface receptor. By using the host cell's genetic material, it replicates its genome to produce viral proteins which are then 'assembled'. The virus then exits the cell through a process called 'budding'.

Antiviral drugs will harness the properties of the viral replication cycle to prevent viral replication from occurring. Table 6.5 summarises the key principles of several antiviral drugs.

**Table 6.5** Antiviral drugs

| Viral infection | Drug name | Mode of drug action |
| --- | --- | --- |
| Human immunodeficiency virus (HIV) | zidovudine | Zidovudine inhibits the action of an enzyme found in HIV, called reverse transcriptase, which is necessary to produce viral DNA and HIV (steps 4–5) |
|  | efavirenz | Efavirenz is a non-competitive inhibitor of HIV-1 reverse transcriptase (step 4) |
|  | enfuvirtide | Enfuvirtide is a fusion inhibitor. It blocks HIV from attaching to the cell surface and entering the host cell (step 2) |
| Hepatitis C | elbasvir | Elbasvir inhibits viral RNA replication and virion assembly (step 4) |
|  | grazoprevir (Zepatier) | Grazoprevir is an inhibitor of a protease enzyme essential for viral replication (steps 4–5) |
| Influenza A and B | oseltamivir | Oseltamivir phosphate is a pro-drug of the active metabolite, oseltamivir carboxylate). The active metabolite is a selective inhibitor of influenza virus enzymes, which are glycoproteins found on the virion surface. These enzymes are necessary for viral entry |
| Human herpes simplex virus (HSV) types I and II and varicella (chickenpox) and herpes zoster (shingles) viral infections | aciclovir | Aciclovir is a direct acting antiviral of the reverse transcriptase inhibitor group, which inhibits viral DNA replication (steps 4–5) |

DNA
virus capsule

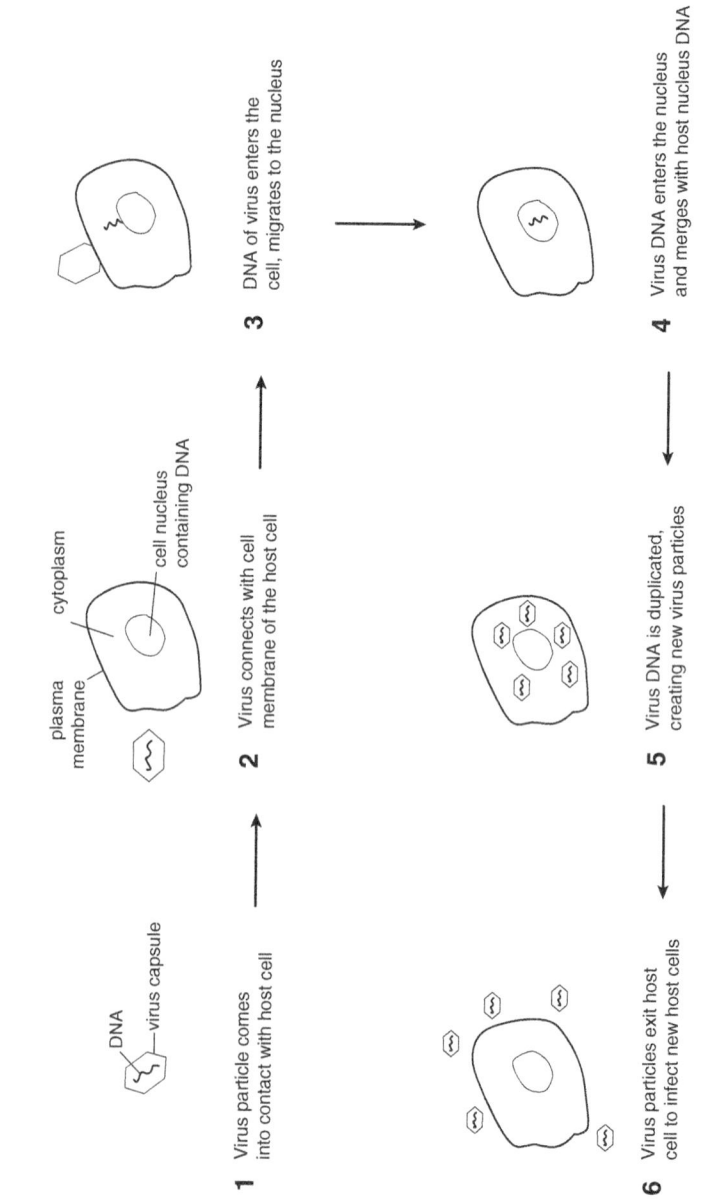

plasma membrane
cytoplasm
cell nucleus containing DNA

1 Virus particle comes into contact with host cell

2 Virus connects with cell membrane of the host cell

3 DNA of virus enters the cell, migrates to the nucleus

4 Virus DNA enters the nucleus and merges with host nucleus DNA

5 Virus DNA is duplicated, creating new virus particles

6 Virus particles exit host cell to infect new host cells

**Figure 6.10** How a virus enters the host cell

## Cancer Pharmacology

There is a wide range of systemic drug treatments which include chemotherapy, immune modulators and targeted biological therapies employed in oncology.

The challenge with traditional cytotoxic agents is that they cannot discriminate between malignant cells and the host cell, resulting in loss of hair follicles, for example. Advances in drug development increasingly target the histology and genotype of the tumour.

Beyond its curative potential, systemic therapy plays a crucial role in increasing overall survival rates among cancer patients. In instances where cure may not be attainable, systemic therapy offers a valuable avenue for palliation allowing some control over disease progression and the alleviation of symptoms, enhancing patients' quality of life. Finally, systemic treatments are used with external treatment as neoadjuvant or induction treatments when local interventions would prove insufficient. Systemic therapies include:

- Chemotherapy (e.g. etoposide, cisplatin)
- Biologic therapies (e.g. interferon)
- Endocrine/hormonal therapy (e.g. tamoxifen)
- Targeted therapy (e.g. tyrosine kinase inhibitors such as gefitinib)
- Proteins demonstrating elevated expression in neoplastic tissues, which offer a strategic focus for therapeutic intervention – for example targeting human epidermal growth factor receptor 2 (HER2) in breast cancer
- Molecular targets which play a fundamental role in the pathogenesis of cancer such as the BCR-ABL fusion protein in chronic myeloid leukemia (CML)
- Targets that lack vital roles in normal tissues and present an opportunity for selective targeting, such as vascular endothelial growth factor (VEGF) in angiogenesis-related cancers
- Targets that can be inhibited pharmacologically, leading to discernible anti-tumour effects and represent a tangible avenue for therapeutic development – for example, the BRAF gene (B-Raf proto-oncogene) in melanoma amongst the population with these specific BRAF mutations

The ideal drug for treating cancer exhibits a high specificity and affinity for its target, ensuring precise interaction with the intended cellular components. This targeted approach is crucial as it minimises adverse effects and enhances the drug's overall efficacy. Upon interacting with its designated target, the drug needs to have potent anti-tumour effects to have a good therapeutic effect. Furthermore, the ideal cancer drug needs to be easily predictable and consistent so that it works similarly in everyone with minimal adjustment to give consistent patient responses to treatment.

## HOW DO CYTOTOXIC DRUGS WORK?

One of the biggest differences between normal cells and cancer cells is that tumour cells have very poor DNA repair mechanisms. This creates a strategic opportunity for targeted cancer therapy. In contrast to normal cells, which possess more efficient repair and replacement mechanisms, tumour cells are more susceptible to the detrimental effects of DNA damage. Intermittent chemotherapy takes advantage of this vulnerability by inducing DNA damage in both normal replicating cells and tumour cells. However, the crucial distinction lies in the different recovery rates between these two cell types. While normal cells can repair and regenerate more quickly, tumor cells experience delayed recovery, providing a therapeutic opportunity for intervention. Chemotherapies may often be used in combination to target different areas of the cell cycle or a particular weakness within the cell cycle of a particular form of cancer (see Figure 6.11 and Table 6.6).

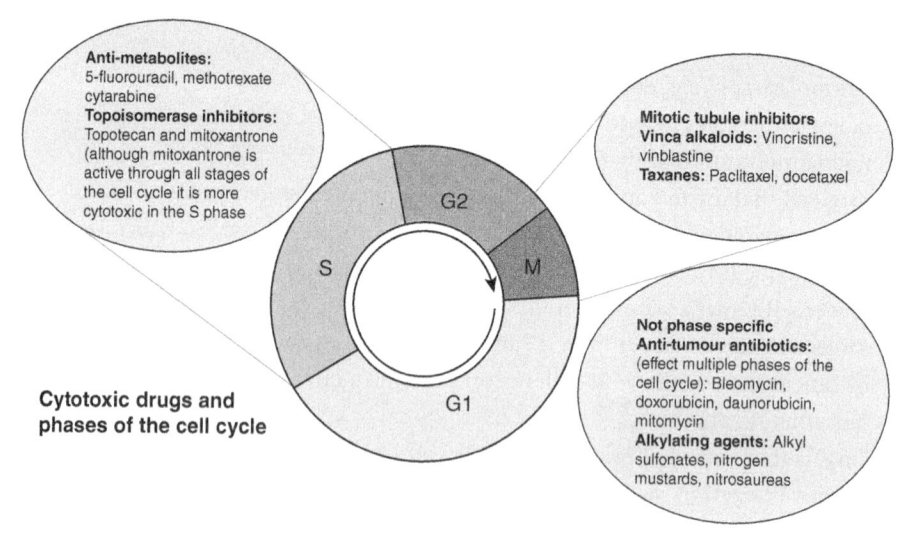

**Figure 6.11** How cytotoxic drugs work

**Table 6.6** Chemotherapy agents

| Chemotherapy agents | Examples |
| --- | --- |
| *Alkylating agents*<br>Directly damage DNA (not phase-specific) | Nitrogen mustards – chlorambucil, cyclophosphamide<br>Nitrosoureas – streptozocin<br>Alkyl sulfonates – busulfan<br>Platiunum group – cisplatin |
| *Antimetabolites*<br>Interfere with DNA and RNA growth (active during S phase of cell cycle) | e.g. 5-fluorouracil<br>Methotrexate<br>Cytarabine |

| | |
|---|---|
| *Anti-tumour antibiotics*<br>Anthracyclines – interfere with enzymes involved in DNA replication | Bleomycin<br>Doxorubicin<br>Daunorubicin |
| *Topoisomerase inhibitors*<br>Interfere with topoisomerase inhibitors which help separate the DNA strands so they can be copied | Topotecan, mitoxantrone |
| *Mitotic inhibitors*<br>Active during M phase | Paclitaxel, docetaxel<br>Vinblastine, vincristine |
| **Immunotherapy**<br>Monoclonal antibodies<br>Non-specific immunotherapies | Rituximab<br>Interleukins – e.g. aldesleukin and interferons |

The induced DNA damage in tumour cells serves as a pivotal mechanism to impede the production of daughter cells or, in some cases, trigger programmed cell death, such as through the induction of apoptosis. This targeted disruption of the cell cycle in tumour cells, coupled with their compromised ability to repair DNA damage efficiently, explains the potential efficacy of intermittent chemotherapy in selectively targeting and inhibiting the growth of cancerous cells. By exploiting these differences in DNA repair mechanisms, therapeutic strategies can be tailored to maximise the impact on tumour cells while minimising adverse effects on normal tissues, contributing to the development of more effective and selective cancer treatments.

In a similar way to antimicrobial resistance, cancer cells too can become resistant to chemotherapy. In antimicrobial resistance, however, the risk is to the general population more than to the individual because microbial diseases are transmitted. In the case of cancer chemotherapy, the risk is to the individual but the way that cancer cells become resistant is like the way bacteria become resistant to antibiotics. This principle also explains why chemotherapy might stop working or that a specific treatment does not give the anticipated results. It also supports the use of combination therapies to treat a cancer as it is less likely that specific tumour cells would be resistant to a combination of two or three chemotherapy drugs. For example, combining cisplatin and 5-fluorouracil involves an alkylating agent to damage DNA and an anti-metabolite to prevent DNA synthesis and repair. This dual approach targets multiple aspects of cancer cell proliferation, reducing the risk of resistance development. There are two primary categories of resistance: primary resistance and secondary resistance.

## Primary Resistance

This occurs when the tumour is not initially sensitive to the selected treatment. Cancer cells may inherently possess characteristics that make them less susceptible to the cytotoxic effects of chemotherapy. The genetic variation in tumours can contribute to this primary resistance, so not all cancer cells will respond uniformly to a given treatment.

## Secondary Resistance

Secondary resistance develops when a tumour, initially responsive to a specific treatment, becomes resistant. Cancer cells arising from mutations can undergo further genetic changes, leading to the development of subpopulations that are resistant to the cytotoxic effects of chemotherapy. These mechanisms of resistance are obvious if you think about it. If a cancer cell changes its cell membrane so that the drug cannot enter then it cannot be killed. Once the drug is inside the cancer cell, the cell could mutate to develop enzymes to break down the drug molecule or have a pump to pump it straight back out. As a couple of final examples, cancer cells could mutate and develop different metabolic pathways to bypass the section of the cell cycle being interrupted, or they could even just become better at repairing DNA.

# FACTORS WHICH AFFECT PHARMACODYNAMICS

Despite understanding the mode of action of a drug, several factors are known to affect this process.

## Age

With advancing age, the number and responsiveness of cell receptors can be affected, which results either in adverse drug responses or in treatment failure. For example, the benzodiazepine group of drugs (e.g. diazepam, lorazepam) act by binding to GABA (gamma-aminobutyric acid) receptors in the brain. The neurotransmitter GABA acts on GABA receptors in the brain to induce sedation and reduce anxiety. With advancing age, the composition and number of GABA receptors declines. This results in GABA receptors becoming more sensitive to the sedating effects of benzodiazepines.

Age-related changes to the cardiovascular system and function result in an increased risk of cardiovascular complications with anaesthetic drugs, which also have an enhanced effect on the older person. Similarly, because age affects cardiovascular and respiratory function in several ways, including the responsiveness of the $\beta$-adrenoreceptors to adrenaline, a drug which acts on these receptors will result in a reduction in response and therefore therapeutic effect.

Whilst growth and the maturity of organs in the neonate and child impact significantly on pharmacokinetics resulting in variability, there is limited data on the pharmacodynamics influences, particularly with respect to the expression and sensitivity of receptors to drugs. As with the older adult, variability in GABA receptor numbers accompanied by differences in the regional blood flow of the brain may alter the brain's responsiveness to central nervous system drugs such as midazolam. Similarly, neonates are more sensitive to neuromuscular blocking agents. Also, due to the paucity of smooth muscle in the bronchial tree, bronchodilators prescribed for the treatment of bronchospasm are ineffective.

## Receptor Activation and Responsivity

The production of cell receptors is genetically determined and therefore their numbers, responsiveness and affinity to the ligand may change over time. For example, it is widely acknowledged that individuals who take the opioid group of drugs (e.g. diamorphine, morphine) over a prolonged period become 'tolerant' to the therapeutic effects and require increased doses to achieve the same level of therapeutic effect. However, tolerance is not the same as an individual's dependency or addiction. The concept of tolerance is highly complex and can vary depending on the specific substance, dosage, duration of exposure and an individual's genetics, physiology and associated pathophysiology. However, understanding the multifaceted nature of tolerance is important for managing it clinically.

Tolerance is defined in two ways:

1. *Innate*: The genetic makeup of the individual may lead to an increased sensitivity or a reduced responsiveness at the receptor level.
2. *Acquired*: Because of increased exposure to the drug, receptor responsiveness is diminished over time, which results in therapeutic failure and the need for increased dosage to achieve the same level of therapeutic effect.

Using the opioid group of drugs as an example, morphine sulphate is an agonist drug which binds to the receptor subtype, the μ-opioid receptor, to produce analgesia and the associated side effect profile. Prolonged stimulation of the μ-opioid receptor by the agonist drug morphine results in a decrease in the expression of the specific receptors with associated desensitisation and degradation of receptors. This is termed 'receptor down-regulation'. This initially results in reduced sensitivity and receptor activation to the ligand or agonist, which results in the need for a greater amount of the agonist to achieve the same level of effect.

In addition, chronic exposure to a drug or substance can lead to changes in gene expression, resulting in increased drug metabolism in the liver or increased synthesis of neurotransmitters that might counteract or enhance the drug in some way.

With morphine or psychoactive drugs chronic exposure to drugs or substances can induce neuroadaptations in the central nervous system, including changes in neurotransmitter release, receptor density and synaptic plasticity. These neuroadaptations can alter the brain's response to the substance, also contributing to tolerance.

Similar changes to the receptor population are seen in the acute withdrawal of the antihypertensive drug clonidine resulting in a rebound hypertensive crisis.

Pathological changes seen in disease, ageing and an individual's genetic makeup will inevitably result in differences seen in an individual's pharmacodynamic response, drug safety profile and therapeutic outcomes.

---

### PAUSE AND REFLECT 6.3

Think about the concept of drug tolerance. Choose a medication you are familiar with and explore how tolerance to this drug can develop. What are the clinical implications of drug tolerance for long-term treatment?

---

## CHAPTER SUMMARY

Chapter 6 has focused on the principles of pharmacodynamics, defined as the mode of action of drugs. Drugs employ a range of principles to exert their therapeutic effect. It is important to understand normal physiological functioning and the pathological changes seen in disease to fully appreciate how drugs act to achieve the desired therapeutic response.

# CASE STUDIES 7
## APPLYING PRINCIPLES TO NURSING PRACTICE

---
### LEARNING OUTCOMES
---

By the end of this chapter, you should be able to:

1. Apply the principles of pharmacokinetics - drug absorption, distribution, metabolism and excretion - and pharmacodynamics to case scenarios.
2. Consider how individual client characteristics, polypharmacy, drug-drug and drug-food interactions can influence pharmacokinetics and pharmacodynamics
3. Explore the role of the health and social care practitioner in the decision-making trail to ensure the safe and therapeutic use of medicines

---

## INTRODUCTION

This chapter presents a range of case studies and related activities, the analysis of which will support and consolidate your learning of the pharmacological concepts in the safe and therapeutic administration and monitoring of drugs in practice.

For each of the case studies presented in this chapter, a client will be introduced in the context of their clinical presentation, past medical history and drug history. Clinical and reflective questions will be asked relating to the presentation of the client, pharmacokinetics and related pharmacodynamics. Please be encouraged to use the preceding chapters and other, external sources to answer the questions before being tempted to review the answers and summary statements.

--- CASE STUDY 7.1 ---

### A Herbal Rejection

Mr Daniel Bortey, a 56-year-old male, underwent a heart transplant due to end-stage heart failure secondary to ischaemic cardiomyopathy. The transplant surgery was successfully

*(Continued)*

performed, and postoperative recovery was uneventful. Mr Bortey was prescribed a regimen of immunosuppressive medications to prevent organ rejection, including ciclosporin 125 mg daily, azathioprine 100 mg daily and prednisolone 10 mg daily. Regular follow-ups were scheduled with the transplant unit to monitor his progress. For the first year post transplant, Mr Bortey's recovery was satisfactory. His ciclosporin concentrations remained within the therapeutic range, and there were no signs of rejection. However, approximately one year post transplant, Mr Bortey began experiencing a decline in mood. Feeling a little low, he sought alternative remedies and visited a local herbal shop. Upon discussing his symptoms, he was recommended St John's Wort, a herbal supplement commonly used for mood enhancement. Over the course of four weeks, he noticed a significant increase in fatigue, which progressively worsened. Concerned about his deteriorating condition, Mr Bortey sought medical advice from his general practitioner (GP). Mr Bortey's GP noted his profound fatigue and promptly referred him to the transplant unit for further assessment. In hospital the transplant team established that there was no infection, but laboratory tests revealed that Mr Bortey's ciclosporin levels were below the target range (50 ng/mL), indicating suboptimal immunosuppression. Additionally, a biopsy of the endomyocardium was performed, which confirmed cellular rejection of the transplanted heart tissue.

## CLINICAL QUESTIONS AND REFLECTIONS

1. What is the significance of monitoring ciclosporin levels in heart transplant recipients, and what is the target therapeutic range?
2. Describe the potential interactions between St John's Wort and ciclosporin. How can this interaction impact immunosuppressive therapy?

## ANSWERS

1. Monitoring ciclosporin levels is crucial to ensure therapeutic efficacy and prevent toxicity. The target therapeutic range for ciclosporin in heart transplant recipients typically falls between 100 and 300 ng/mL.
2. St John's Wort is known to induce cytochrome P450 enzymes, which can accelerate the metabolism of ciclosporin, leading to reduced plasma concentrations and potentially suboptimal immunosuppression. Induction of liver enzymes does not happen straight away and instead takes place over several weeks. It is important to remember that some drug interactions or adverse effects happen weeks later following the commencement of treatment.

## SUMMARY AND CONCLUSION

In response to the findings, Mr Bortey's immunosuppressive regimen was adjusted. The dose of ciclosporin was increased, and additional monitoring was commenced to ensure optimal drug levels. Azathioprine and prednisolone dosages were also reassessed to address the rejection episode. Mr Bortey was educated about the potential interactions between herbal supplements, particularly St John's Wort, and prescribed medications. He was advised to discontinue the use of herbal products. Following the adjustments in his medication regimen and cessation of St John's Wort, Mr Bortey's fatigue gradually improved, and subsequent follow-ups indicated stabilisation of his immunosuppressive levels. Repeat biopsy showed resolution of cellular rejection, and his overall mood also improved with appropriate support and counselling.

This case explains the importance of awareness regarding potential interactions between herbal supplements and prescribed medications, particularly in the context of organ transplantation and immunosuppressive therapy. Healthcare providers should actively inquire about the use of alternative remedies and provide comprehensive education to patients to mitigate risks and ensure optimal outcomes post transplantation. Vigilant monitoring and timely intervention are crucial in managing complications and promoting the long-term success of organ transplantation.

---------- CASE STUDY 7.2 ----------

### A Poor Choice

Oleksandr, a 10-year-old boy, presented to A&E (accident and emergency) with complaints of severe headache and fever. He had been experiencing these symptoms for the past two days and his parents decided to seek medical attention due to increasing concern. Upon evaluation, Oleksandr was diagnosed with acute tonsillitis and prescribed codeine to manage his headache and associated discomfort. He was prescribed 15-30 mg every four to six hours as needed for pain based on his body mass. Shortly after receiving the medication, Oleksandr exhibited signs of respiratory depression, including shallow breathing and decreased oxygen saturation levels. Recognising the seriousness of the situation, the medical team intervened promptly to address the respiratory depression and prevent further complications. Thanks to the timely administration of naloxone and appropriate medical intervention, Oleksandr's respiratory depression resolved quickly and his vital signs stabilised.

## TREATMENT AND OUTCOME

Oleksandr's respiratory depression was promptly managed with the administration of naloxone, which reversed the opioid effects. He was closely monitored for any recurrence of symptoms and was discharged once his vital signs stabilised. His caregivers were educated about the risks of codeine in children, and alternative pain management strategies were discussed with the family.

## CLINICAL QUESTIONS AND REFLECTIONS

1   What are the current recommendations regarding the use of codeine in paediatric patients, and what factors contribute to the increased risk of respiratory depression in this population?

2. How does codeine exert its analgesic effects, and what are the potential adverse effects associated with its use in paediatric patients?
3. What are the signs and symptoms of opioid-induced respiratory depression, and how should healthcare providers monitor paediatric patients for these complications when prescribing codeine?
4. What is the mechanism of action of naloxone, and how does it reverse opioid-induced respiratory depression in paediatric patients?
5. Why is codeine more of a risk in children than adults?

## ANSWERS

1. Current recommendations advise against the use of codeine in paediatric patients due to the increased risk of respiratory depression and other adverse effects, particularly in those with ultra-rapid metaboliser phenotypes of CYP2D6. Factors contributing to the increased risk include variable metabolism rates, immature drug-metabolising enzymes, and individual genetic variations affecting codeine metabolism.
2. Codeine is a prodrug that requires conversion to its active form morphine by the liver enzyme CYP2D6 for its analgesic effects. Adverse effects associated with codeine use in paediatric patients include respiratory depression, sedation, nausea, vomiting, constipation and potential for addiction or dependence.
3. Healthcare providers should monitor paediatric patients who have inappropriately received codeine for signs of opioid-induced respiratory depression, including decreased respiratory rate, shallow breathing, confusion, lethargy and cyanosis. Close observation is particularly important in younger children and those with underlying respiratory conditions.
4. Naloxone is an opioid antagonist that works by competitively binding to opioid receptors, displacing opioids such as codeine and reversing their effects on the central nervous system. Naloxone rapidly restores normal respiratory function and reverses the symptoms of opioid-induced respiratory depression.
5. Children exhibit considerable variability in drug metabolism, especially in the context of codeine, which requires conversion to its active metabolite morphine by the liver enzyme CYP2D6. Some children may have ultra-rapid metaboliser phenotypes, resulting in rapid and excessive conversion of codeine to morphine, leading to higher morphine concentrations and increased risk of respiratory depression. This is coupled with the fact that children generally exhibit increased sensitivity to the central nervous system effects of opioids compared to adults and will lead to increased risk of respiratory depression in children. Factors such as immature blood–brain barrier function and differences in opioid receptor density and distribution may also contribute to children's heightened sensitivity to opioid-induced respiratory depression.

## CASE STUDY 7.3

### Does Dose Matter?

Mr Jamal Thompson, a 58-year-old man, presented to the emergency department with complaints of chest pain and dyspnoea. He has a past medical history significant for hypertension and type 2 diabetes mellitus. Mr Thompson was prescribed aspirin dispersible 75 mg and paroxetine 20 mg daily. Despite being prescribed 75 mg aspirin post ST-elevation myocardial infarction (STEMI), Mr Thompson decided to self-medicate with 2 x 300 mg aspirin tablets, believing that a higher dose would provide better protection against further cardiac events. Many months passed, during which time, Mr Thompson continued to take the higher dose of aspirin. Mr Thompson also experienced heartburn and gastrointestinal discomfort shortly after increasing his aspirin dosage. On evaluation, Mr Thompson was found to have evidence of ongoing myocardial ischemia and that he had also developed a bleeding ulcer, probably as a result of the higher-dose aspirin.

## CLINICAL QUESTIONS AND REFLECTIONS

1. How does aspirin exert its antiplatelet effects, and what is the mechanism behind its action?
2. Why is low-dose aspirin preferred for antiplatelet therapy post-STEMI, and how does it help reduce adverse effects?
3. Why doesn't high-dose aspirin have the same antiplatelet effects as low-dose aspirin?
4. Why do aspirin and other NSAIDs cause gastrointestinal bleeding?
5. Can SSRIs like paroxetine increase or decrease the risk of bleeding in patients taking aspirin and how?

## ANSWERS

1. Aspirin exerts its antiplatelet effects by irreversibly inhibiting the enzyme cyclooxygenase-1 (COX-1), which is responsible for the conversion of arachidonic acid into thromboxane A2, a potent platelet activator. By inhibiting COX-1, aspirin blocks the synthesis of thromboxane A2, thereby reducing platelet aggregation and thrombus formation. The irreversible inhibition of COX-1 by aspirin means that the effects on platelets persist for the lifespan of the platelet (about 7–10 days), as new platelets are unable to synthesise thromboxane A2. This mechanism provides long-lasting antiplatelet effects even after aspirin has been metabolised and cleared from the body.
2. Low-dose aspirin (typically 75–100mg) is preferred for antiplatelet therapy post-STEMI because it achieves sufficient inhibition of platelet function while

minimising the risk of adverse effects, particularly gastrointestinal bleeding. At low doses, aspirin is absorbed in the stomach and meets platelets primarily in the hepatic portal vein before undergoing first-pass metabolism in the liver. This allows for localised inhibition of platelet COX-1 activity, reducing systemic exposure and potential adverse effects.

3   It is possible that aspirin also has effects on the vasculature. For example, chronic exposure to aspirin could impair endothelial nitric oxide (NO) synthesis, which plays a crucial role in maintaining vascular homeostasis and regulating vascular tone. Endothelial dysfunction may predispose blood vessels to increased platelet adhesion and thrombus formation, cancelling the effect on platelets to an extent.

4   Whilst there can be direct mucosal injury from aspirin and NSAIDs because they are acidic solids, most of the effects of aspirin and NSAIDs are systemic, occurring once the drugs have entered the circulation. NSAIDs, including aspirin, exert their therapeutic effects by inhibiting the activity of cyclooxygenase enzymes, particularly COX-1 and COX-2. COX enzymes play a crucial role in the synthesis of prostaglandins, which are lipid mediators involved in maintaining the integrity of the gastric mucosa, regulating gastric blood flow and promoting mucus secretion and bicarbonate production. All these things protect the stomach mucosa from acid erosion. By inhibiting COX enzymes, NSAIDs reduce the production of prostaglandins, leading to decreased mucosal protection and increased susceptibility to injury. Additionally, prostaglandins help maintain mucosal blood flow, which is essential for providing oxygen and nutrients to the gastric epithelial cells. All these factors make the stomach mucosa more susceptible to damage from stomach acid and less able to repair, leading to ulceration and possibly bleeding.

5   The mechanism behind this interaction involves the inhibition of platelet function. Platelets are blood cells responsible for clotting and they play a crucial role in preventing excessive bleeding. Serotonin is involved in platelet aggregation, which is the process of platelets clumping together to form a clot. SSRIs can interfere with this process by inhibiting the uptake of serotonin into platelets, leading to decreased platelet aggregation and potentially increased bleeding risk.

## SUMMARY AND CONCLUSION

This case highlights the dangers of self-adjusting prescribed medication doses, particularly with drugs like aspirin that have a narrow therapeutic margin. It underscores the need for patient education on appropriate medication use and the importance of consulting healthcare providers before making any changes to prescribed regimens.

## CASE STUDY 7.4

### Don't Take Other People's Medication

Mei Lin, an 80-year-old woman, has a complex medical history and is currently managing multiple chronic conditions. She resides at home and relies on support from family members and district nurses for her healthcare needs. Mei Lin takes several medications regularly, including digoxin for heart failure, furosemide for oedema and ibuprofen for an ankle sprain given to her by a relative who had them in the house for something else. Mei Lin's mobility is limited, and she avoids drinking excess fluids due to the inconvenience of frequent trips to the toilet. During a visit by district nurses to change a dressing on a pressure sore, Mei Lin exhibits concerning symptoms of abdominal pain, nausea, vomiting and visual disturbances. She describes seeing a yellow glow around her room lamp. An ambulance is called to take Mei Lin to hospital.

## CLINICAL QUESTIONS AND REFLECTIONS

1. How do the pharmacological mechanisms of digoxin, furosemide and ibuprofen interact in the context of polypharmacy, and what are the potential consequences of their combined use in an elderly patient?
2. What are the pharmacokinetic and pharmacodynamic considerations when prescribing digoxin, furosemide and ibuprofen in an elderly patient with limited mobility and potential renal impairment?
3. How does digoxin toxicity manifest clinically and what factors contribute to the increased risk of toxicity in elderly patients, particularly in the presence of polypharmacy and renal function decline?
4. What are the potential drug–drug interactions between digoxin, furosemide and ibuprofen, and how do these interactions contribute to the development of adverse effects such as digoxin toxicity?
5. What is the phenomenon of the yellow hue around lights related to?

## ANSWERS

1. Digoxin is a cardiac glycoside that increases myocardial contractility and reduces heart rate, while furosemide is a loop diuretic that promotes diuresis by inhibiting sodium and chloride reabsorption in the kidney. Ibuprofen is a non-steroidal anti-inflammatory drug (NSAID) with analgesic, anti-inflammatory and antipyretic properties. In polypharmacy, the concurrent use of these medications can lead to electrolyte imbalances, particularly hypokalaemia induced by furosemide, which can exacerbate the risk of digoxin toxicity.
2. Elderly patients such as Mei Lin may experience altered drug metabolism, reduced renal function and increased sensitivity to medications due to age-related changes

in physiology. Digoxin is primarily eliminated via renal excretion, raising concerns for drug accumulation and toxicity in the setting of renal impairment. Additionally, furosemide-induced electrolyte disturbances, particularly hypokalaemia, can potentiate the cardiotoxic effects of digoxin. Ibuprofen can alter renal function due to the non-selective inhibition of prostaglandins which in the renal system act to keep renal tubules patent. A reduction in renal function would increase the accumulation of digoxin.

3  Digoxin toxicity can manifest clinically with gastrointestinal symptoms such as nausea, vomiting and abdominal pain, as well as neurological symptoms including confusion, visual disturbances (e.g. xanthopsia) and cardiac arrhythmias. Elderly patients are at increased risk of toxicity due to age-related changes in drug metabolism, reduced renal function and increased susceptibility to drug interactions.

4  Digoxin, furosemide and ibuprofen can interact pharmacokinetically and pharmacodynamically, potentially leading to adverse effects and toxicity. Furosemide-induced hypokalaemia can pharmacodynamically increase digoxin toxicity by enhancing its cardiac effects, while ibuprofen can pharmacokinetically reduce renal function leading to increased digoxin concentrations and enhanced pharmacological effects.

5  The yellow hue or visual disturbance described by the patient, known as xanthopsia, is a notable clinical manifestation of digoxin toxicity. Xanthopsia is characterised by the perception of yellow or greenish-yellow visual disturbances, often described as a yellow halo or glow around objects. This phenomenon occurs because of the effects of digoxin on the visual system, particularly its ability to alter colour perception. The mechanism underlying digoxin-induced xanthopsia is not fully understood but is believed to involve alterations in retinal sensitivity to light and changes in colour perception. Digoxin may interfere with the function of retinal cone cells, which are responsible for colour vision, leading to a distortion in colour perception and the perception of a yellowish tint or halo around objects.

## SUMMARY AND CONCLUSION

Digoxin primarily exerts its pharmacological effects by inhibiting the sodium–potassium ATPase pump (Na+/K+-ATPase) in myocardial cells. This inhibition leads to an increase in intracellular sodium concentration and a subsequent decrease in intracellular potassium concentration. As a result, there is an indirect inhibition of the sodium–calcium exchanger (NCX), leading to an increase in intracellular calcium concentration. Hypokalaemia exacerbates digoxin toxicity by further reducing intracellular potassium levels. Potassium is crucial for maintaining the resting membrane potential and normalising the duration of the action potential in cardiac cells. Low potassium levels prolong the duration of the action potential, predisposing myocardial cells to increased intracellular calcium concentrations, which can lead to abnormal cardiac rhythms and contractility. The combination of digoxin-induced inhibition of Na+/K+-ATPase and hypokalaemia-induced alterations in potassium homeostasis synergistically affects cardiac electrophysiology. This synergistic effect results in enhanced intracellular calcium concentrations and increased myocardial contractility, leading to a higher risk of adverse cardiac events such as arrhythmias, conduction disturbances and ventricular fibrillation.

Recognising the potential for digoxin toxicity exacerbated by polypharmacy and renal function decline due to NSAID use, the district nurses promptly notify Mei Lin's primary care physician. Mei Lin is advised to discontinue ibuprofen immediately and arrangements are made for urgent blood tests to assess her renal function, electrolyte levels and digoxin concentration.

Blood tests reveal elevated serum digoxin levels and evidence of renal impairment, confirming the diagnosis of digoxin toxicity. Mei Lin's digoxin dose is adjusted and she is closely monitored for resolution of symptoms and improvement in renal function. With appropriate management and discontinuation of ibuprofen, Mei Lin's symptoms gradually subside and she experiences no further episodes of digoxin toxicity.

This case explains the importance of careful medication management, especially in elderly patients with multiple comorbidities. Polypharmacy, combined with factors such as limited mobility, dehydration and impaired renal function, can significantly increase the risk of adverse drug reactions and drug interactions. Healthcare providers must remain vigilant and consider the potential risks and benefits of each medication in the context of the individual patient's medical history and circumstances. Regular medication reviews, close monitoring of symptoms and proactive communication among healthcare providers, patients and caregivers are essential for optimising medication safety and minimising the risk of adverse drug events in elderly patients with complex medication regimens.

## CASE STUDY 7.5

### A Change in Diet

Ana Dominguez, a 42-year-old female with a history of bipolar disorder, prescribed lithium carbonate, was admitted to the hospital because she had entered a period of dangerously poor mental health and, in addition, had not been caring for herself well. Further investigation revealed that Ana had not been taking her medication regimen, resulting in low lithium levels 0.2 mmol/L (0.5-1.2 mmol/L). During hospitalisation, her lithium levels were stabilised within the therapeutic range (0.5-1.2 mmol/L), and her diet was improved to high-fibre, low-fat and low-salt intake. Upon discharge, she returned home but reverted to her previous dietary habits. After a few weeks, however, she was re-admitted through A&E with signs and symptoms of lithium toxicity and her lithium levels were dangerously high at 1.9 mmol/L (0.5-1.2 mmol/L).

## TREATMENT AND OUTCOME

Ana was promptly treated for lithium toxicity with intravenous fluids and discontinuation of lithium therapy. Close monitoring of lithium levels and supportive care were provided until her symptoms resolved and lithium levels returned to the therapeutic range. Upon discharge, Ana was counselled on the importance of medication adherence and dietary modifications to prevent recurrence of lithium toxicity.

## CLINICAL QUESTIONS AND REFLECTIONS

1. What are the common signs and symptoms of lithium toxicity?
2. How does poor dietary habits, particularly high-salt intake, contribute to lithium toxicity in patients taking lithium carbonate?
3. What groups are at higher risk of lithium toxicity?
4. What monitoring should be done for patients taking lithium carbonate to prevent and detect toxicity?

## ANSWERS

1. Common signs and symptoms of lithium toxicity include confusion, tremors, nausea, vomiting, diarrhoea, muscle weakness, blurred vision, and seizures.
2. Poor dietary habits, particularly high-salt intake, can lead to lithium toxicity by competitively inhibiting renal excretion of lithium salts, resulting in their accumulation in the body. Due to it being a simple ionic salt, liver enzymes cannot metabolise lithium and so elimination is entirely dependent on renal excretion.
3. Elderly individuals are at increased risk of lithium toxicity due to age-related changes in kidney function, which can impair lithium clearance, leading to accumulation and toxicity. Similarly, patients with impaired renal function, whether from age, chronic kidney disease, or other factors, may experience decreased lithium clearance, predisposing them to toxicity. Dehydrated individuals are also at risk, as dehydration can reduce renal perfusion and impair lithium excretion, increasing the likelihood of lithium accumulation and toxicity. Additionally, certain medications, including diuretics, NSAIDs, ACE inhibitors, and SSRIs, can interfere with lithium clearance, elevating lithium levels and toxicity risk. As well as high sodium levels causing accumulation, low sodium levels (hyponatremia) can also lead to increased reabsorption of lithium in the kidneys, contributing to higher lithium levels and heightened toxicity risk. Acute illnesses or conditions affecting fluid balance, like vomiting, diarrhoea, or severe infections, can alter renal function and hydration status, potentially leading to lithium toxicity.

4   Monitoring parameters for patients taking lithium carbonate include serum lithium levels, renal function tests, thyroid function tests, and assessment of symptoms indicative of lithium toxicity.

## SUMMARY AND CONCLUSION

As Ana resumed her high-salt diet, renal excretion of sodium chloride competed with lithium salts for excretion, leading to the accumulation of lithium levels in the blood. Consequently, the patient presented to the hospital again with signs and symptoms of lithium toxicity, including confusion, tremors, and nausea. Laboratory investigations revealed dangerously high blood levels of lithium, necessitating readmission for urgent management. This case highlights the critical importance of medication adherence and dietary modifications in patients receiving lithium therapy for bipolar disorder. It explains the potential consequences of non-compliance with medication regimens and the impact of dietary habits on medication effectiveness and toxicity. Multidisciplinary interventions addressing medication adherence, dietary habits and social support are essential in the comprehensive management of patients with bipolar disorder receiving lithium therapy.

---

### PAUSE AND REFLECT 7.1

Consider the importance of patient adherence to medication regimens. Reflect on the barriers that might prevent a patient from taking their medication as prescribed. What strategies can healthcare professionals use to improve adherence?

---

### CASE STUDY 7.6

### Acute Dystonic Reaction

Aisha, a 16-year-old female, was planning a trip with her family. Concerned about travel sickness, she visited her family physician who prescribed metoclopramide, a common medication used to alleviate nausea and vomiting associated with motion sickness. Aisha took the medication as directed, hoping for a comfortable journey. However, shortly after ingestion, she began experiencing unexpected symptoms. Soon after taking the metoclopramide, Aisha developed distressing facial and skeletal muscle spasms, along with a sensation of her eyes rolling upwards uncontrollably. These symptoms of course caused Aisha and her family significant distress and anxiety. Recognising the severity of her symptoms, they quickly went to A&E.

## CLINICAL QUESTIONS AND REFLECTIONS

1. What is the mechanism of action of metoclopramide and how does it relate to the development of acute dystonic reactions?
2. Why is this more prevalent in young women?
3. What are the typical clinical manifestations of acute dystonic reactions and how do they differ from other neurological conditions?
4. Why is procyclidine chosen as the treatment of choice for acute dystonic reactions caused by metoclopramide?
5. What are the potential complications of untreated acute dystonic reactions and how can prompt intervention improve patient outcomes?

## ANSWERS

1. Metoclopramide is a dopamine receptor antagonist that primarily acts on D2 receptors in the brain. In some cases, excessive dopamine blockade can lead to dysregulation of motor control pathways, resulting in acute dystonic reactions characterised by involuntary muscle contractions.
2. We are not sure why this is more prevalent in young women, and the answer is likely to be a combination of factors. For example, it is thought that hormonal fluctuations during puberty and menstrual cycles may influence the sensitivity of dopamine receptors in the brain. Oestrogen has been shown to modulate dopamine activity, potentially increasing the susceptibility of young women to adverse reactions involving dopamine antagonists like metoclopramide. It may also be that receptor density may be higher in young women and therefore systems affected by dopamine antagonism may be more profoundly affected. Finally, young people, including young women in their teens, may experience higher levels of stress, anxiety and emotional distress compared to other demographic groups. Stress and psychological factors have been linked to the development of acute dystonic reactions and other extrapyramidal symptoms, potentially exacerbating the effects of dopamine antagonists like metoclopramide. However, none of this has been established with certainty and whatever the cause the MHRA/CHM should never be a first-line choice and only in certain cases as second line.
3. Clinical manifestations of acute dystonic reactions often include facial grimacing, tongue protrusion, neck stiffness and abnormal eye movements such as oculogyric crises. These symptoms are typically sudden in onset and may mimic other neurological conditions, but they are distinct in their association with recent medication administration, such as metoclopramide.
4. Procyclidine is an anticholinergic medication that antagonises muscarinic receptors in the brain, counteracting the excessive dopamine blockade induced by metoclopramide. By restoring the balance between dopamine and acetylcholine, procyclidine effectively alleviates the symptoms of acute dystonic reactions.

5   Untreated acute dystonic reactions can lead to prolonged discomfort, distress and potential complications such as dehydration due to difficulty swallowing or respiratory compromise in severe cases. Prompt intervention with medications like procyclidine can effectively alleviate symptoms, prevent complications and improve overall patient outcomes.

## SUMMARY AND CONCLUSION

This case emphasises the potential for rare but serious side effects of common medications like metoclopramide, particularly in susceptible populations such as young women. It also highlights the importance of prompt recognition and treatment of acute dystonic reactions to prevent the distress these reactions can cause.

--- CASE STUDY 7.7 ---

### An Incidental Finding

Mr Giovanni Rossi, a 60-year-old man, presented to A&E with rectal bleeding. He is known to be a smoker and has a history of deep vein thrombosis (DVT) for which he has been taking warfarin for the past couple of months. Despite having a chaotic life and often forgetting to take his medications, Mr Rossi has been consistent with his warfarin regimen. However, he has been trying to improve his lifestyle by eating more healthily and reducing his smoking. He has been finding it easier to lose weight lately and lost 6 kg over the last month, which he attributes to a reduced appetite.

Upon examination, Mr Rossi was found to have bright red rectal bleeding, which was determined to be caused by haemorrhoids. The bleeding was exacerbated by his anticoagulant therapy with warfarin. Further evaluation revealed a significantly elevated INR (International Normalised Ratio) of 5.

Additional investigations were carried out to explore the underlying cause of Mr Rossi's weight loss and revealed advanced lung cancer. The weight loss, initially attributed to reduced appetite, was indicative of an underlying malignancy. The rectal bleeding, exacerbated by his anticoagulant therapy, was attributed to haemorrhoids but warranted close monitoring due to his high INR. Mr Rossi was admitted for further management, including stabilisation of his INR, symptomatic management of haemorrhoids and initiation of palliative care for his advanced lung cancer.

## CLINICAL QUESTIONS AND REFLECTIONS

1   What are the key pharmacokinetic parameters of warfarin?
2   How is Mr Rossi's profound and sudden weight loss related to his elevated INR?
3   Why was Mr Rossi given warfarin instead of the first-line DOAC?

## ANSWERS

1. Warfarin is highly bound to albumin in the plasma. Warfarin is extensively metabolised by the liver, primarily through the **cytochrome P450 enzyme system**, specifically CYP2C9. Genetic variations in CYP2C9 can affect warfarin metabolism and dosage requirements. Warfarin and its metabolites are excreted mainly through the kidneys, with a long half-life of about 20 to 60 hours.
2. Mr Rossi's profound and sudden weight loss can significantly affect the pharmacokinetics of warfarin. Warfarin is highly protein-bound, and changes in body weight can raise the concentration of free (unbound) drug in the bloodstream. With weight loss, the volume of distribution decreases, leading to higher concentrations of free warfarin, which can result in increased anticoagulant effects and an elevated INR. Additionally, weight loss may affect the patient's dietary habits and metabolism, potentially impacting warfarin metabolism and clearance.
3. Mr Rossi's erratic medication adherence and chaotic lifestyle may have raised concerns about his ability to comply with the strict dosing regimens associated with DOACs. This is important with DOACs because they have relatively short half-lives. The longer half-life of warfarin means that this was an optional second-line choice for the patient.

## SUMMARY AND CONCLUSION

This case demonstrates the interconnected nature of a patient's symptoms and the importance of comprehensive evaluation, even when symptoms initially appear unrelated. It also highlights the impact of changes such as weight loss, on drug pharmacokinetics and the need for monitoring of patients on anticoagulant therapy.

─────────── CASE STUDY 7.8 ───────────

### Pharmacokinetic Interactions

Name: Mr John Smith
Age: 65
Diagnosis: Chronic obstructive pulmonary disease (COPD)
Medical History: COPD exacerbations, hypertension
Smoking Status: Active smoker for 30+ years

### Case Presentation

Mr John Smith, a 65-year-old man diagnosed with COPD, presented to his GP complaining of worsening dyspnoea and increased coughing. He had a long history of smoking, approximately one pack per day for over 30 years. His previous exacerbations of COPD were managed with short-acting bronchodilators and corticosteroids. Due to the frequency of exacerbations, his physician decided to initiate theophylline therapy to help manage his symptoms.

## Initial Treatment

Theophylline was initiated at a low dose of 200 mg extended release once daily of a specific brand, with plans for dose adjustment based on therapeutic drug monitoring (TDM).

Mr Smith was advised on the importance of adhering to the medication regimen and the potential adverse effects associated with theophylline, especially considering its narrow therapeutic range.

## Therapeutic Drug Monitoring

Blood samples were collected periodically to monitor serum theophylline levels.

Initial TDM showed that Mr Smith's serum theophylline levels were within the therapeutic range (5-15 µg/mL) with the prescribed dose.

## Follow-Up Appointment

During a follow-up visit, Mr Smith's GP told Mr Smith that his bloods 'looked good' and emphasised the importance of smoking cessation in managing his COPD and slowing down its progression. Mr Smith then decided to quit smoking and was referred to the smoking-cessation advisor. There Mr Smith was provided with resources and support to aid in smoking cessation.

## Critical Incident

After four weeks Mr Smith started experiencing symptoms of theophylline toxicity, including nausea, vomiting, headache and palpitations. Further TDM revealed significantly elevated serum theophylline levels (>20 µg/mL), indicating toxicity. Theophylline therapy was immediately discontinued and supportive measures were initiated to manage the adverse effects.

## Outcome and Final Follow-Up

With the cessation of theophylline therapy and supportive management, Mr Smith's symptoms of toxicity gradually resolved. Alternative treatment options for managing his COPD were explored, considering the risks associated with theophylline therapy. Mr Smith was closely monitored for any recurrence of COPD symptoms and adverse effects related to theophylline.

## TREATMENT AND OUTCOME

Mr. Smith's theophylline therapy was discontinued, and supportive management, including IV fluids, was provided to alleviate his symptoms of toxicity. Smoking cessation support continued, and alternative treatments for COPD were initiated. Mr. Smith's symptoms resolved, and a tailored COPD management plan was developed to prevent further complications.

## CLINICAL QUESTIONS AND REFLECTION

1. Why did this happen? Think about how Mr Smith stopping smoking may have caused an issue.
2. What factors contribute to the decision to initiate theophylline therapy in a COPD patient like Mr Smith?
3. Describe the mechanism of action of theophylline and its role in managing COPD symptoms.
4. Why is therapeutic drug monitoring (TDM) important for patients receiving theophylline therapy?
5. Discuss the concept of a 'narrow therapeutic range' and its implications for medication management.
6. How does smoking affect the metabolism of theophylline, and what are the potential consequences for patients like Mr Smith?
7. What steps should healthcare professionals take to support smoking cessation in COPD patients receiving theophylline therapy?
8. What are the signs and symptoms of theophylline toxicity, and how should healthcare providers manage a patient experiencing these symptoms?
9. What alternative treatment options could be considered for managing COPD in patients who develop theophylline toxicity?
10. Why does the case study mention prescribing the drug by brand?

## ANSWERS

1. Mr Smith successfully quit smoking, which led to the removal of the induction of theophylline metabolism caused by nicotine. As a result, serum theophylline levels began to rise gradually despite no change in the dosage regimen. This case explains the importance of therapeutic drug monitoring and individualised treatment in patients receiving medications with a narrow therapeutic range, such as theophylline. Healthcare professionals should be vigilant in assessing and managing potential drug interactions, especially when lifestyle changes, such as smoking cessation, are implemented. Collaboration between healthcare providers and patients is crucial for optimising treatment outcomes and minimising the risk of adverse effects.

2. The decision to initiate theophylline therapy in a COPD patient like Mr Smith is typically based on factors such as the frequency and severity of exacerbations, inadequate response to other bronchodilators or corticosteroids, and the need for additional long-term maintenance therapy to improve lung function and symptoms.

3. Theophylline is a bronchodilator that works by relaxing the smooth muscles in the airways, thereby improving airflow, and reducing symptoms of COPD such as dyspnoea and coughing. The action of theophylline is complex, but its primary mechanisms of action involve its effects on adenosine receptors and inhibition of phosphodiesterase enzymes. Theophylline antagonises adenosine receptors, particularly the A1 and A2 subtypes. Adenosine, when it binds to its receptors, causes bronchoconstriction and promotes inflammation in the airways. By blocking these receptors, theophylline prevents this bronchoconstriction by adenosine, leading to bronchodilation and improved airflow in the lungs. Theophylline also inhibits phosphodiesterase enzymes, primarily phosphodiesterase type III and to a lesser extent type IV. These enzymes normally break down cyclic adenosine monophosphate (cAMP) and cyclic guanosine monophosphate (cGMP), which are important intracellular signalling molecules involved in smooth muscle relaxation. By inhibiting phosphodiesterase, theophylline increases the levels of cAMP and cGMP, leading to relaxation of bronchial smooth muscles and further bronchodilation. That said, theophylline probably also has several other effects including stimulation of respiratory drive and anti-inflammatory properties.

4. Therapeutic drug monitoring (TDM) is important for patients receiving theophylline therapy because it has a narrow therapeutic range, meaning that the difference between the minimum effective concentration and the toxic concentration is small. TDM helps ensure that serum theophylline levels are within the therapeutic range to optimise efficacy and minimise the risk of toxicity.

5. A 'narrow therapeutic range' refers to the narrow margin between the minimum effective concentration and the toxic concentration of a drug. In the case of theophylline, maintaining serum levels within this range is crucial for achieving therapeutic effects while avoiding adverse effects.

6. Smoking induces the metabolism of theophylline by increasing the activity of cytochrome P450 enzymes, particularly CYP1A2. This leads to accelerated clearance of theophylline from the body, potentially resulting in sub-therapeutic serum levels and decreased efficacy of the medication.

7. Healthcare professionals should provide comprehensive support for smoking cessation, including counselling, behavioural interventions, pharmacotherapy (e.g. nicotine replacement therapy or prescription medications), and referral to smoking cessation programs or support groups. Emphasising the importance of smoking cessation in improving COPD outcomes and optimising theophylline therapy can motivate patients like Mr Smith to quit smoking.

8  Signs and symptoms of theophylline toxicity include nausea, vomiting, headache, palpitations, arrhythmias, seizures and potentially life-threatening cardiac events. Management of theophylline toxicity involves discontinuation of the medication, supportive care (e.g. IV fluids, anti-emetics) and, in severe cases, administration of activated charcoal or haemodialysis to enhance elimination of the drug.

9  Alternative treatment options for managing COPD in patients who develop theophylline toxicity may include other bronchodilators (e.g. long-acting beta-agonists, anticholinergics), inhaled corticosteroids or biologic therapies such as monoclonal antibodies targeting specific inflammatory pathways. In this case theophylline could have been used but monitoring should have been much more frequent and rate of reduction in nicotine carefully considered and monitored.

10 Prescribing theophylline by brand ensures consistency in dosing and bioavailability, which is crucial for maintaining therapeutic levels within the narrow range required. Different brands of theophylline may have different bioavailabilities and/or dose regimens.

---

## CASE STUDY 7.9

### A Hidden Danger Unmasked

Mrs Anika Patel, a 35-year-old woman, recently married. Since she married, she has been taking the combined oral contraceptive pill for one month. She visited her GP complaining of symptoms suggestive of a urinary tract infection (UTI). Upon consultation, Mrs Patel was prescribed nitrofurantoin 100 mg twice daily for a week to treat her UTI. Mrs Patel went on a holiday to Cornwall during June where she was exposed to hot and sunny weather. However, after three days of nitrofurantoin treatment, she experienced a sudden onset of distressing symptoms and sought emergency medical attention at the A&E department.

Mrs Patel presented with pain in the back, abdomen and legs, vomiting, a degree of confusion, dark brown or reddish urine and skin blistering upon sunlight exposure. Upon admission to A&E, Mrs Patel underwent various diagnostic tests to determine the underlying cause of her symptoms. There was concern that her symptoms were indicative of a worsening infection or sepsis. However, her temperature was normal and although some aspects of her presentation were indicative of sepsis, this didn't fit the whole clinical picture. Blood tests revealed an ongoing infection (although resolving, as indicated by relatively normal white blood cell count), slightly elevated blood pressure, and normal renal and liver function. Stool samples and urine were collected for further analysis and all her existing medicines were stopped and she was started on antibiotic cefuroxime 750 mg every six to eight hours.

## TREATMENT AND OUTCOME

Mrs. Patel was treated with supportive measures, including hydration and discontinuation of triggering medications, which alleviated her symptoms. Her diagnosis of acute porphyria was confirmed through genetic testing, and she received counselling on avoiding known triggers and adjusting her lifestyle to prevent future attacks.

## CLINICAL QUESTIONS AND REFLECTIONS

1. What is acute porphyria?
2. What are the typical symptoms of acute porphyria, and how do they correlate with the symptoms presented by Mrs Patel?
3. Why is sunlight exposure a concern for patients with acute porphyria?
4. How might nitrofurantoin and the combined oral contraceptive pill contribute to the development of acute porphyria in susceptible individuals?
5. How can pharmacogenomic testing aid in the management of patients with acute porphyria?
6. What alternative antibiotic options could have been considered for treating Mrs Patel's urinary tract infection to avoid exacerbating her acute porphyria?
7. How are acute attacks of porphyria typically treated?

## ANSWERS

1. Acute porphyria refers to a group of rare inherited metabolic disorders characterised by deficiencies in enzymes involved in haem biosynthesis, leading to the accumulation in the body of haem precursors called porphyrins. The four main types of acute porphyria include acute intermittent porphyria (AIP), variegate porphyria (VP), hereditary coproporphyria (HCP) and ALAD-deficiency porphyria (ADP). These disorders typically manifest with episodic attacks of symptoms that can affect various body systems, including the nervous system, gastrointestinal tract and skin. Some people remain asymptomatic throughout their life and some people may only have one episode, but others can have more. The onset and severity of symptoms can be triggered by various factors, including certain medications, hormonal changes, alcohol consumption, fasting and stress. Management of acute porphyria primarily involves symptom relief, avoiding triggers and preventing complications. Treatment during acute attacks often includes intravenous administration of glucose and hemin to suppress haem synthesis and alleviate symptoms. Early diagnosis and proper management are crucial to prevent complications and improve the quality of life for individuals with acute porphyria. Genetic counselling and testing can help identify individuals at risk and guide treatment strategies.

2. Typical symptoms of acute porphyria include abdominal pain, neuropathic pain, vomiting, confusion and dark urine. Mrs Patel's presentation aligns with these symptoms, indicating a possible diagnosis of acute porphyria.
3. Sunlight exposure can exacerbate symptoms of acute porphyria by triggering the production of reactive oxygen species in the skin, leading to further accumulation of porphyrins, and causing skin blistering, photosensitivity and pain.
4. Nitrofurantoin is known to induce hepatic enzymes involved in haem synthesis, potentially exacerbating porphyrin accumulation and precipitating acute porphyria attacks in individuals with an underlying genetic predisposition. COCPs containing oestrogen can increase the synthesis of hepatic enzymes involved in haem synthesis, potentially exacerbating porphyrin accumulation and contributing to the manifestation of acute porphyria symptoms in susceptible individuals.
5. Pharmacogenomic testing can identify genetic variations in enzymes involved in haem synthesis, helping clinicians predict individual susceptibility to drug-induced porphyria and tailor medication regimens accordingly to minimise the risk of triggering acute attacks.
6. Local guidelines vary and the advice on safe/unsafe drugs in acute porphyria can be found in the British National Formulary but alternative antibiotic options for treating urinary tract infections in patients with acute porphyria may include trimethoprim-sulfamethoxazole, fosfomycin or ciprofloxacin as these agents are less likely to induce hepatic enzymes involved in haem synthesis. Mrs Patel was put on an antibiotic to treat sepsis due to uncertainty for treatment and stopping her drugs will have helped resolve the porphyria.
7. Hydration with intravenous fluids helps to correct electrolyte imbalances and maintain renal function. Intravenous glucose infusion can suppress hepatic haem synthesis, reducing the production and release of porphyrins. Hemin, a haem precursor, is administered intravenously to individuals experiencing severe attacks to reduce the activity of delta-aminolaevulinic acid synthase (ALAS), an enzyme involved in haem synthesis. This helps to alleviate symptoms and shorten the duration of attacks.

## SUMMARY AND CONCLUSION

Mrs Patel underwent genetic testing, confirming the diagnosis of acute porphyria. This information guided her long-term management plan. Her healthcare team provided ongoing education and counselling on lifestyle modifications, including dietary recommendations (e.g. regular meals, avoidance of fasting), medication management and contraception choices. Mrs Patel received regular follow-up appointments with her healthcare provider to monitor her. Genetic counselling was offered to Mrs Patel and her family members to assess the inheritance pattern of acute porphyria and provide guidance on family planning and reproductive options.

## CASE STUDY 7.10

### Lithium Therapy: All Is Not Equal

Mrs Johnson, a 60-year-old female, presents with a viral infection causing a very sore throat, which makes swallowing hard solids difficult. She reports no other significant symptoms and is otherwise well hydrated and able to maintain sufficient oral intake. Mrs Johnson has been stable on lithium carbonate tablets at a dose of 400 mg daily, with a consistent lithium serum level of 1 mmol/l. She has been managing her mental health condition effectively with this treatment regimen. Concerned about Mrs Johnson's ability to continue taking her lithium tablets due to her current difficulty swallowing, her GP decides to switch her medication to lithium citrate liquid. The GP prescribes 4 mL daily of lithium citrate 520 mg/5 mL for a duration of two weeks.

After a week, the district nurse visits Mrs Johnson to take blood samples and perform basic observations. Mrs Johnson appears to be uncharacteristically unwell during the visit, but it is attributed to her ongoing viral infection, which is otherwise resolving. The lab results reveal a significant drop in Mrs Johnson's lithium serum level to 0.6 mmol/L, indicating a sub-therapeutic concentration. The drop in lithium levels correlates with the switch from lithium carbonate tablets to lithium citrate liquid even though 4 mL of liquid is the same dose as Mrs Johnson had been taking in tablet form previously. Recognising the importance of maintaining therapeutic lithium levels for Mrs Johnson's mental health stability, the GP advises Mrs Johnson to resume her lithium carbonate tablets upon completion of the liquid prescription.

Mrs Johnson complies with her GP's instructions and resumes her lithium carbonate tablets. After another week, her lithium levels increase to 0.9 mmol/L, indicating a return to therapeutic levels. Mrs Johnson reports feeling much better, both physically and mentally, with her symptoms of the viral infection subsiding and her mental health stabilised.

## CLINICAL QUESTIONS AND REFLECTIONS

1. Why was the GP concerned about the drug's effectiveness if Mrs Johnson was unable to take her medication correctly. Link this to the pharmacology of lithium.
2. Why was the GP concerned to make sure that the patient was not dehydrated? Again, link this to the pharmacology of lithium.
3. Define the term bioavailability.
4. Use the British National Formulary (BNF) or Electronic Medicines Compendium (EMC) medicines to observe the difference between the bioavailability of the tablet form of lithium and the liquid form.
5. Conclude what would have been a more appropriate dose for switching to the liquid form of the drug for this patient.

## ANSWERS

1. The GP was concerned about the effectiveness of Mrs Johnson's medication because her inability to take it correctly could lead to fluctuations in serum lithium levels, affecting its pharmacological action. Lithium has a narrow therapeutic index, meaning small changes in serum levels can result in significant clinical effects. If Mrs Johnson couldn't take her medication as prescribed, it could lead to suboptimal drug levels, increasing the risk of relapse of her mental health condition. This concern is directly linked to the pharmacology of lithium, as its therapeutic effects are closely tied to maintaining stable serum levels within the therapeutic range.

2. The GP was concerned about ensuring Mrs Johnson was not dehydrated because lithium's pharmacokinetics are influenced by hydration status. Lithium is predominantly eliminated by the kidneys and dehydration can lead to decreased renal function, impairing lithium excretion. This can result in elevated serum lithium levels, potentially leading to lithium toxicity. Therefore, maintaining adequate hydration is essential to support renal function and prevent lithium toxicity, highlighting the pharmacological relationship between hydration status and lithium metabolism.

3. Bioavailability refers to the proportion of a drug that enters systemic circulation unchanged after administration and is available to produce a pharmacological effect. It is a measure of the rate and extent to which a drug reaches the systemic circulation and is typically expressed as a percentage.

4. According to the BNF or EMC, the bioavailability of lithium carbonate tablets is approximately 80–100%, while the bioavailability of lithium citrate liquid is around 30–70%. This indicates that the tablet form of lithium has higher bioavailability compared to the liquid form.

5. Considering the difference in bioavailability between the tablet and liquid forms of lithium, a more appropriate dose for switching to the liquid form for Mrs Johnson would be to adjust the dose of lithium citrate liquid to compensate for its lower bioavailability. Since the liquid form has a bioavailability of approximately 30–70% compared to the tablet form, a higher dose of lithium citrate liquid may be necessary to achieve equivalent serum lithium levels. Therefore, the GP may consider prescribing a higher dose of lithium citrate liquid, perhaps 8 ml, to ensure Mrs Johnson maintains therapeutic serum levels during the transition from lithium carbonate tablets.

---------- CASE STUDY 7.11 ----------

### Induction into a Withdrawal Situation

Paul Davison, a 20-year-old male, presented to the drug clinic seeking assistance with his heroin addiction and concerns about HIV exposure. Paul reported a history of heroin use for the past two years, and he recently discovered he had been exposed to HIV through shared needles. Motivated to address both his addiction and potential HIV infection, Paul expressed a desire to quit heroin and undergo appropriate treatment.

CASE STUDIES | 163

Given Paul's heroin addiction, the healthcare team initiated methadone maintenance therapy to assist with opioid withdrawal and addiction management. In adherence to typical starting regimens in the UK, Paul was prescribed an initial dose of methadone at 30 mg daily, which was to be administered under supervised conditions at the clinic.

A week later Paul was reviewed, and his test results came back positive, confirming the presence of the virus.

Following the confirmation of HIV infection, Paul was started on antiretroviral therapy to manage his HIV. The prescribed regimen included tenofovir alafenamide (TAF), emtricitabine (FTC), and darunavir. Despite the initiation of methadone therapy, Paul reported ongoing cravings and withdrawal symptoms. As a result, the healthcare team decided to increase his methadone dose slightly to 40 mg daily to better manage his symptoms.

Unfortunately, despite the adjustments to his methadone regimen, Paul experienced a relapse in heroin use a couple of weeks later. He reported severe withdrawal symptoms and difficulty maintaining abstinence. Recognising the challenges Paul faced in managing his addiction, the healthcare team conducted a thorough reassessment of his treatment plan.

## CLINICAL QUESTIONS AND REFLECTIONS

1. Describe the clinical manifestations of sub-therapeutic methadone levels in a patient undergoing opioid maintenance therapy.
2. Explain the concept of drug metabolism induction.
3. Explore how this relates to methadone and darunavir interactions.
4. What factors contribute to the long half-life of methadone, and how does this pharmacokinetic property influence its dosing regimen?
5. What alternative approaches could be considered for managing Paul's opioid withdrawal symptoms in the context of reduced methadone levels due to darunavir-induced metabolism?

## ANSWERS

1. Sub-therapeutic methadone levels can lead to opioid withdrawal symptoms in patients undergoing opioid maintenance therapy. These symptoms may include anxiety, agitation, sweating, nausea, vomiting, diarrhoea, muscle aches and drug cravings. Patients may experience a worsening of their addiction symptoms, leading to difficulty in maintaining abstinence from illicit opioids.
2. Drug metabolism induction occurs when a drug increases the activity of enzymes responsible for its own metabolism. This process leads to accelerated metabolism and clearance of the drug from the body, resulting in reduced plasma concentrations over time. Drug metabolism induction often involves the activation of specific enzymes, such as cytochrome P450 (CYP) enzymes in the liver, which are responsible for metabolising many drugs.

3   Methadone induces its own metabolism by increasing the activity of hepatic enzymes, including CYP3A4, which metabolise methadone. This auto-induction results in accelerated clearance of methadone from the body, leading to lower plasma concentrations over time. The implications of this phenomenon for clinical use include the potential for reduced efficacy of methadone therapy and the need for dose adjustments to maintain therapeutic plasma levels. Similarly, darunavir, an HIV protease inhibitor, can induce the metabolism of methadone by increasing the activity of CYP3A4 enzymes. Together these inductions lead to accelerated clearance of methadone, resulting in reduced plasma levels and potential sub-therapeutic concentrations.

4   The long half-life of methadone is attributed to several factors, including its high lipid solubility, extensive tissue distribution and slow metabolism. Methadone is metabolised primarily in the liver, but it has a prolonged elimination half-life ranging from 15 to 60 hours or longer. This pharmacokinetic property allows for once-daily dosing in opioid maintenance therapy and provides sustained opioid receptor occupancy, reducing the frequency of opioid withdrawal symptoms. But it also results in challenges when altering doses and initiating therapy.

5   Alternative approaches for managing Paul's opioid withdrawal symptoms may include increasing the dose of methadone to compensate for the accelerated clearance due to darunavir-induced metabolism. Additionally, switching to a different opioid maintenance therapy such as buprenorphine or incorporating adjunctive medications or psychosocial interventions may be considered to address his symptoms and support his recovery from opioid addiction. Close monitoring and collaboration between healthcare providers are essential to optimise treatment outcomes in such cases.

Considering Paul's relapse, the healthcare team re-evaluated his treatment plan and explored alternative approaches to address his heroin addiction. This included considerations for increasing his methadone dose further, transitioning to buprenorphine-based therapy, or integrating additional psychosocial support services to enhance his treatment outcomes.

## CHAPTER SUMMARY

Drugs are prescribed to manage physiological derangements by either preventing or treating disease and supporting homeostatic mechanisms amongst other functions. It is therefore essential that medicine management is safe and therapeutic.

Chapter 7, the final chapter of the book, has presented several clinical case studies which raise concerns about the safety and therapeutic efficacy of drugs and which require clinical management. The case studies individually and collectively were designed to support your learning and professional application of key pharmacological principles discussed in previous chapters. They were also intended to encourage you to consider more deeply the role that the practitioner plays in medicine management.

# BIBLIOGRAPHY

British Medical Association and Royal Pharmaceutical Society (2024). *British National Formulary (BNF)*. https://bnf.nice.org.uk (Accessed 15 November 2024).

Dean, L. and Kane, M. (2025) Codeine Therapy and CYP2D6 Genotype. In V.M. Pratt, S.A. Scott, M. Pirmohamed (Eds.) *Medical Genetics Summaries* [Internet]. Bethesda (MD): National Center for Biotechnology Information (US). https://www.ncbi.nlm.nih.gov/books/NBK100662/ (Accessed 11 February 2025).

EMC (2024). *EMC: Electronic Medicines Compendium*. www.medicines.org.uk/emc (Accessed 15 November 2024).

European Parliament and Council of the European Union (2010). Directive 2010/84/EU of the European Parliament and of the Council of 15 December 2010 amending, as regards pharmacovigilance, Directive 2001/83/EC on the Community code relating to medicinal products for human use. *Official Journal of the European Union*, L 348, 74–99. https://eur-lex.europa.eu/legal-content/EN/TXT/?uri=CELEX%3A32010L0084 (Accessed 15 November 2024).

Jung Kim, H. and Hyun Park, S. (2014) Sciatic nerve injection injury. *Journal of International Medical Research*, 42(4): 887–897. doi:10.1177/0300060514531924

Kaestli, L.Z., Wasilewski-Rasca, A.F., Bonnabry, P., Vogt-Ferrier, N. (2008) Use of Transdermal Drug Formulations in the Elderly. *Drugs Aging*, 25(4): 269–80. doi: 10.2165/00002512-200825040-00001.

Lin SK. (2022) Racial/Ethnic Differences in the Pharmacokinetics of Antipsychotics: Focusing on East Asians. *Journal Personalized Medicine*, 12(9): 1362. doi.org/10.3390/jpm12091362

Medicines and Healthcare products Regulatory Agency (MHRA) (2024). *Medicines and Healthcare products Regulatory Agency*. www.gov.uk/government/organisations/medicines-and-healthcare-products-regulatory-agency (Accessed 15 November 2024).

National Institute for Health and Care Excellence (NICE) (2024). *NICE Guidelines*. www.nice.org.uk/guidance (Accessed 15 November 2024).

Nursing and Midwifery Council (NMC) (2018) *Future Nurse: Standards of Proficiency for Registered Nurses*. London: NMC. https://www.nmc.org.uk/globalassets/sitedocuments/education-standards/future-nurse-proficiencies.pdf (Accessed 15 November 2024).

Rajman, I., Knapp, L., Morgan, T. and Masimirembwa, C. (2017) African Genetic Diversity: Implications for Cytochrome P450-mediated Drug Metabolism and Drug Development. *EBioMedicine*, 17: 67–74.

World Health Organization (WHO) (2002). *Safety of Medicines: A Guide to Detecting and Reporting Adverse Drug Reactions*. www.who.int/publications/i/item/WHO-EDM-QSM-2002-2 (Accessed 15 November 2024).

Zhong, Z., Hou, J., Li, B., Zhang, Q., Liu, S., Li, C., Liu, Z., Yang, M., Zhong, W., Zhao, P. (2017) Analysis of CYP2C19 Genetic Polymorphism in a Large Ethnic Hakka Population in Southern China. *Med Sci Monit*, 23: 6186–6192. doi: 10.12659/msm.905337.

# GLOSSARY

**Absorption**: The first stage of pharmacokinetics and is the process of the drug moving from the site of administration to the bloodstream.

**Acid**: A chemical substance that donates hydrogen ions when dissolved in water. The higher the concentration of hydrogen ions, the more acidic the solution.

**Active transport**: The process of moving substances into, out of and between cells, using energy.

**Affinity**: The strength of attraction between a drug and its receptor on the cell's surface.

**Agonist**: A substance which activates a physiological response when combined with a receptor.

**Allosteric modulator**: A substance that binds to a receptor to change that receptor's response to stimuli.

**Anaesthetic**: A drug used to cause a temporary loss of awareness or sensation. There are two groups: general anaesthetics used to induce a reversible loss of consciousness (i.e. during surgery) and local anaesthetics which provide a reversible loss of sedation and are limited to a region of the body.

**Analgesic**: The group of drugs that are used to relieve or control pain. They are sometimes referred to as pain killers or pain relievers.

**Angiotensin-converting enzyme inhibitors (ACEIs)**: A class of drug that blocks the production of angiotensin II, a substance that narrows blood vessels. By blocking, this drug helps to widen blood vessels and thus reduces blood pressure.

**Antacid**: A drug that neutralises stomach acid and so can be effective when experiencing acid reflux or 'heartburn' or to relieve the symptoms of a gastric ulcer.

**Antagonist**: A substance that binds to the receptor and stops that receptor from producing a response.

**Anti-arrhythmic**: A drug that helps prevent and treat abnormal heart rhythms. They may stop irregular and extra impulses or prevent fast electrical impulses from travelling along the heart tissue.

**Anticoagulant**: A drug that prevents or reduces the clotting of blood, commonly known as blood thinners, and reduces the risks of strokes, pulmonary embolisms and myocardial infarctions.

**Antidepressant**: A drug used to regulate mood by adjusting neurotransmitter levels to alleviate symptoms of depression and other mental health conditions.

**Antihistamine**: A drug that blocks the effect of histamine in the body. Histamines are chemicals that help get rid of allergens and toxins as part of the immune system and can cause inflammation, mucous, sneezing and itching. By blocking histamine, antihistamines can prevent the symptoms of allergies.

**Antimicrobial**: A drug that kills or prevents the growth of microorganisms. Antimicrobial drugs include antibiotics, antivirals and anti-fungal drugs.

**Anxiolytics**: A drug that reduces anxiety and related psychological symptoms. They reduce nervous system activity.

**Atom**: The fundamental building block of matter; everything is made of atoms.

**Base (alkaline)**: A substance that forms hydroxide ions when dissolved in water.

**Beta blocker**: A drug that blocks the action of adrenaline on beta receptors in blood vessels and in the heart. This reduces the force of heart contractions and slows down the heart rate.

**Bioavailability**: The amount of drug that reaches the systemic circulation. When a drug is administered via the intravenous or intra-arterial routes, the drug has 100% bioavailability as it directly enters the bloodstream.

**Biotransformation**: See *Metabolism*.

**Bradycardia**: This relates to a low heart rate. For adults it is usually considered to be a heart rate under 60 beats per minute.

**Buccal**: This means relating to the cheek. A drug that is administered via the buccal route is placed between the gum and cheek and then dissolves and is absorbed into the bloodstream.

**Calcium channel blocker**: A drug that targets calcium channels in cell membranes and prevents the entry of calcium ions into cells, particularly in heart and smooth muscle cells. Calcium channel blockers help reduce blood pressure by widening the blood vessels (*vasodilation*).

**Cell**: A cell is considered the basic building block of all living organisms. There are single-cell organisms such as bacteria and multi-cellular organisms such as animals and plants.

**Chemoreceptor**: Receptors that detect changes in the chemical composition of the blood and other bodily fluids and play a vital part in homeostasis.

**Compound:** A substance that is made from more than one element.

**Conjugation**: During conjugation reactions, a drug or its metabolites are chemically modified to form larger and/or more water-soluble compounds, facilitating their excretion from the body and limiting their systemic distribution.

**Corticosteroids**: Drugs that resemble cortisol, a hormone that is produced by our body's adrenal glands. They have anti-inflammatory properties and are used to treat conditions such as asthma, lupus, eczema and inflammatory bowel disease.

**Cytochrome P450 enzyme system**: A group of enzymes found in the liver that are vital in the metabolism of *endogenous* (naturally occurring) and *exogenous* (external) compounds. They are involved in Phase I reactions.

**Cytotoxic**: Cytotoxic means something that harms or kills cells. Cytotoxic drugs are used to treat cancer and some *autoimmune* diseases by stopping the growth or function of abnormal or harmful cells.

**Diffusion**: Diffusion is the movement of molecules from a region of higher concentration to that of a lower concentration and is important in the transport of substances in and out of cells.

**Distribution**: The second stage of pharmacokinetics and is the process by which medication is *dispersed* throughout the body from the bloodstream to various tissues and organs in the body.

**Diuretic**: Drugs that increase the amount of water and salt excreted from the body as urine. They are often used to treat high blood pressure, heart failure and other conditions.

**Efficacy** (drug efficacy): The ability of a drug to produce a biological effect once it binds to a receptor.

**Emollients**: Products that hydrate the skin by providing a protective layer to keep in moisture and are used to prevent and treat skin dryness. They are found in creams, lotions, moisturizers and ointments.

**Endocytosis**: The process of actively transporting molecules into a cell by engulfing them with its membrane, used when molecules cannot pass through the membrane passively.

**Endogenous**: Developing or originating within an organism or part of an organism. It refers to something that is produced within the body.

**Enteral**: Enteral refers to the intestines. It means by way of or passing through the intestine, either naturally via the mouth and oesophagus, or through an artificial opening such as a gastrostomy.

**Entero-hepatic recycling**: A process (also known as enterohepatic circulation) in which certain substances are transported between the liver and the intestines. It is important in maintaining bile acid levels and absorption of nutrients and applies to drugs.

**Enzyme**: A protein molecule found in cells that speeds up chemical reactions in the body without being altered in the process, allowing it to be used repeatedly.

**Excretion**: The fourth and final stage of pharmacokinetics and is the process by which the body eliminates the drug.

**Exocytosis**: The opposite of endocytosis, where vesicles containing molecules are moved to the cell membrane where they fuse with the membrane and are secreted into the extracellular environment. It is a form of bulk transport.

**Exogenous**: Originating or produced from outside a cell, tissue or organism.

**Filtration**: Filtration is a process used to separate solids (undissolved particles) from liquids. For example, renal filtration is a process in which the blood is filtered by the glomerulus of the kidney so that essential substances can be selectively reabsorbed.

**First-pass metabolism**: A pharmacological phenomenon in which a drug undergoes metabolism at a specific location in the body, predominantly the liver. The first-pass effect decreases the drug's concentration upon reaching systemic circulation or its site of action.

**Half-life**: The length of time required for the concentration of a drug to decrease to half its starting dose in the body.

**Homeostasis**: A self-regulating process by which biological systems maintain stability, adjusting to conditions that are optimal for survival – for example, the regulation of body temperature.

**Hydrolysis**: A chemical reaction in which one substance reacts with water to produce another.

**Hydrophilic**: The ability of a chemical compound to be mixed with or dissolved in water. A hydrophilic substance has a strong affinity for water.

**Hypertensive**: Refers to raised arterial blood pressure.

**Hypotension**: Refers to low arterial blood pressure.

**Immunosuppressant**: A drug that is used to suppress or reduce the strength of the immune system. They prevent the body's immune system from attacking healthy cells. They can help prevent organ transplant rejection and treat autoimmune disorders.

**Intramuscular**: Refers to being situated in, occurring in, or administered by entering a muscle. An intramuscular injection involves a needle being passed deep into the muscle and fluid delivered to that muscle.

**Intravenous**: Refers to being situated, performed or occurring within or entering by way of a vein.

**Ion**: An ion is a charged particle. It is an atom or molecule that has gained or lost an electron, giving it either a positive or negative electrical charge.

**Laxative**: A drug that increases stool frequency or eases of passage of the stool. It either increases water content in the stool or accelerates bowel transit.

**Ligand**: A ligand is any molecule or atom that binds reversibly to its target receptor.

**Lipophilic**: The ability of a chemical compound to dissolve in lipids and non-polar solvents. Lipophilic substances are attracted to lipids.

**Metabolism**: The third stage of pharmacokinetics. It is the process of breaking down a drug by the body, so it is ready for excretion. It is also known as *biotransformation*.

**Metabolite**: An intermediate or end product of metabolism.

**Molecule**: Molecules are two or more atoms that are chemically bound together.

**Nitrates:** Nitrates are a class of drugs that cause vasodilation by donating nitric oxide (NO) e.g. glyceral trinitrate (GTN). Nitrates dilate venous vessels, coronary arteries and small arterioles, allowing blood to flow more easily thus reducing the amount of work required by the heart.

**Nomenclature**: A system for naming things, especially in science, such as drugs in pharmacology.

**NSAID**: Non-steroidal anti-inflammatory drugs are drugs that reduce pain and inflammation. They work by blocking enzymes which are responsible for producing prostaglandins.

**Opioid**: A group of pain-relieving drugs that attach to opioid receptors in brain cells, blocking pain messages.

**Osmosis**: The spontaneous movement of solvent molecules from an area of low solute concentration to one of high solute concentration through a semi-permeable membrane, in order to equalise their concentrations on both sides of the membrane.

**Oxidation**: An important process in metabolism. It is a chemical reaction resulting in the addition of oxygen and/or the removal of hydrogen. This increases the drug's water solubility and is therefore more likely to be excreted.

**Parenteral**: Refers to treatments or substances that are administered outside the digestive system. For example, it includes drugs that are injected into tissue, muscles or veins rather than given orally.

**Perfusion**: The passage of blood or fluid through the blood vessels to organs or tissue, especially the passage of blood through the lung tissue to pick up oxygen from the air in the alveoli.

**pH**: pH is the acidity or basicity of an aqueous or other liquid solution. It refers to the concentration of hydrogen ions and is denoted by numbers between 0 and 14.

**Pharmacodynamics**: The effects of the drug on the body at a molecular level – that is, how the drug acts to prevent or manage disease and the related signs and symptoms.

**Pharmacogenetics**: Also *pharmacogenomics*, this is the study of how our genes influence our response to medications. It explores how genetic differences can affect the way our bodies process specific drugs.

**Pharmacokinetics**: The study of drug movement through the body or how the body affects the drug.

**Pharmacology**: The study of drugs and their effects on the body.

**Phospholipid**: A type of lipid molecule that has fatty acid tails which are hydrophobic and a phosphate head, which is hydrophilic, attached to a glycerol molecule. Phospholipids are the main component of the cell membrane.

**Polar**: A polar molecule is one whose distribution of electrons between its bonded atoms is uneven. *Polarity* is a description of how different the electrical poles of a molecule are. If they are very different it is considered to be a highly polar molecule.

**Potency**: The potency of a drug is the amount of drug needed to produce a specific biological response. A drug that is more potent will need less of the drug to produce a response.

**Pro-drug**: A drug that is pharmacologically inactive and becomes pharmacologically active following metabolism.

**Proton-pump inhibitors**: Proton pump inhibitors (PPIs) are drugs that decrease the production of stomach acid by irreversibly blocking the proton pump. They are commonly used to treat conditions such as chronic acid reflux and stomach ulcers.

**Receptor**: Receptors are usually glycoproteins found in cell membranes that recognise and bind to ligands such as drugs, neurotransmitters, hormones and growth factors. When a ligand binds to a receptor, it initiates a change in the receptor protein, leading to a series of reactions inside the cell resulting in biological responses.

**Renal clearance**: The rate at which a substance is removed from the blood plasma by the kidneys.

**Selectivity**: Refers to a drug's strong preference for its intended target over other targets.

**Semi-permeable**: This refers to the ability to allow some liquids and gases to pass through it but not others. It is like a selective gateway. The cell membrane is semi-permeable.

**Solute**: A substance that is dissolved in a solvent.

**Solvent:** A substance that dissolves a solute, resulting in a solution.

**Specificity**: How a drug only reacts with its intended target. This is different from selectivity which ensures it does so preferentially among potential targets.

**SSRIs**: Selective serotonin re-uptake inhibitors (SSRIs) are drugs that are typically used as antidepressants in the treatment of depression and other psychological conditions.

**Subcutaneous**: Situated or placed under the skin.

**Sublingual**: Refers to something that is situated or administered under the tongue.

**Substrate**: The material that an enzyme (a chemical produced by living cells) acts on to produce a chemical reaction.

**Sub-therapeutic**: Refers to a drug concentration that is too low to produce the intended medical effect.

**Tachycardia**: Refers to an increased heart rate, usually over 100 beats per minute in an adult.

**Therapeutic index**: The therapeutic ratio measures the safety of a drug. It compares the amount of drug needed to cause toxicity with the amount required to produce the desired therapeutic effect. In other words, it assesses the margin of safety between the effective dose and the toxic dose.

**Therapeutic window**: Refers to the range of drug dosages or concentrations in a bodily system that provides safe and effective therapy. Within this window, the drug achieves its desired effect without causing toxicity.

**Topical**: The application of medication directly to a specific area of the body with the intention of providing a therapeutic effect at that site. Usual topical locations are the skin, ears and eyes.

**Toxicity** (drug toxicity): Refers to how poisonous or harmful a substance can be. It happens when a person accumulates too much of a prescription drug in their bloodstream, leading to adverse side effects.

**Transdermal**: A route of administration where active ingredients are delivered across the skin for systemic distribution.

**Volume of distribution**: The theoretical volume needed to contain the total amount of a drug at the same concentration in the blood plasma. Essentially, it's a measure of how extensively a drug distributes into body tissues rather than remaining in the plasma.

# INDEX

Note: Page numbers followed by f indicate figures; those followed by t indicate tables.

acetylcholine, 123
acetylcholinesterase, 16
acetylsalicylic acid, 104
aciclovir, 133t
acid–base imbalances, 9
acid labile, 40
acids, 9
acne, 53
acrolein, 97
active transport, 13, 22, 22f
acute dystonic reaction, 151–153
acute porphyria, 158–160
acute tonsillitis, 143
adenosine, 92, 157
adenosine triphosphate (ATP), 13, 24
adrenaline, 122, 124
adverse drug reaction (ADR), 115–116
affinity, 73, 125
agonist drug, 119–120, 124t, 124f
albumin, 72, 74, 75
alcohol, 91, 109
alcohol dehydrogenase (ADH), 109
alkaline drugs, 104
allosteric modulator, 125
alpha 1-acid glycoproteins, 72, 75
alprazolam, 120
aminoglycoside antibiotics, 105
amiodarone, 95, 126
amylase, 15
anaesthetics, 9
analgesics, 64
angiotensin-converting enzyme inhibitors (ACEIs), 96, 129–130
angiotensin I/angiotensin II, 129–130
antacids, 39
antagonists, 71, 122–124, 124f, 124t
antibacterial drugs, 131–132
antibiotics, 45
anticholinesterases, 131
anticoagulant drugs, 56, 154
antidepressants, 85, 127, 127f
antihistamines, 64
antimicrobial resistance, 40, 137
antimuscarinic agent, 123
antithrombin, 56
antiviral drugs, 132–133, 133t

arachidonic acid metabolism pathways, 130f
arthritis, 107
ascorbic acid, 35
aspirin, 104, 126t, 130, 145–146
atenolol, 47t, 93
atoms, 6
atracurium, 123
autocrine signalling, 24
azathioprine, 85, 142

bactericidal drugs, 132
bacteriostatic drugs, 132
bacterium, 131–132, 132f
baroreceptors, 5, 6f
bases (alkali), 9
BCG vaccine, 58
BCRP (breast cancer resistance protein), 70
benzodiazepines, 45, 50, 120, 121, 125, 138
benzoyl peroxide, 53
benzylpenicillin, 71
β-carboline compound, 121
beta-adrenergic receptors, 115
beta-blockers, 64, 115, 122
bicarbonate, 14–15
bile, 37, 80
bilirubin, 37, 81
bioavailability, 35, 46–48, 47t, 162
bioequivalent, 48
biotransformation, 79, 82
blood–brain barrier (BBB), 69–72
blood pressure, homeostatic control of, 5–6
brand name, 2
breast milk, 110
breathalyser tests, 109
British Approved Names (BAN), 2
bronchoconstriction, 115
Brunner's glands, 36
buccal and sublingual routes, of drug administration, 48–50, 49f
'budding', 133
buffers, 14
bulk transport, 23f
buprenorphine, 164

calcium, 7, 14
calcium channel blocker, 128

calcium chelation, example of, 41f
calcium ions, 27
cancer pharmacology, 135
captopril, 96, 129
cardiac disease, 88
carrier proteins/pumps, 22, 22f, 127–129
case studies
    acute dystonic reaction, 151–153
    acute porphyria, 158–160
    codeine use in paediatric patients, 143–144
    dangers of self-adjusting prescribed medication doses, 145–146
    digoxin toxicity risk, in elderly patients, 147–149
    herbal supplements and prescribed medications, interactions between, 141–143
    incidental finding, 153–154
    induction into withdrawal situation, 162–164
    lithium therapy, 161–162
    lithium toxicity, and high-salt intake, 149–151
    pharmacokinetic interactions, 154–158
catalysts, 15
caudate lobe, 80
cefuroxime, 158
celecoxib, 130
cell membranes, 13, 14f, 116
    active transport, 22
    bulk transport, 23
    diffusion, 20
    filtration, 22
    osmosis, 20–21
    transport of substances across, 20–23
cell receptors, 117f, 139
cells, 3, 12
    autocrine signalling, 24
    endocrine signalling, 25
    four phases of cell cycle, 27, 28f
    functions of, 23–27
    important parts of, 17f
    juxtacrine, 24–25
    life cycle of, 27, 28f
    paracrine signalling, 25
    sending and receiving of signals, 24
    structure and function of, 16–19
    transduction pathways, 26–27
    types of chemical signalling, 25f
centrioles, 18
cerebrospinal fluid, 12
channel-linked receptors, 117t
chelation, 41
chemoreceptors, 5
chemotherapy agents, 136–137t
chloramphenicol, 42, 86
chloride, 14

chlorpromazine, 75
cholecystokinin, 35
chromium (Cr), 7t
chronic kidney disease (CKD), 107
ciclosporin, 142
ciprofloxacin, 42, 106, 160
circulatory shock, 57
cisplatin, 137
clarithromycin, 90
clopidogrel, 96
clozapine, 89
cobalt (Co), 7, 7t
codeine, 84, 96, 143–144
coeliac disease, 41
cofactor, 16
colon, 44–45
    anatomy, 44f
    primary functions, 44
combination therapy, 128
communication, cell, 24
competitive (reversible) antagonism, 122
compounds, 6, 8
conductivity, 23
control centres, in brainstem, 5
copper (Cu), 7t
corneocytes, 51
corticosteroids, 52–53
covalency, 8
CR (controlled release), 43
curare, 123
*Cutibacterium acnes*, 53
cyclic adenosine monophosphate (cAMP), 27, 157
cyclic guanosine monophosphate (cGMP), 157
cyclo-oxygenase (COX-1 and COX-2), inhibition of, 130, 145, 146
cyclophosphamide, 97
CYP1A2, 83, 87, 88, 89, 90t, 157
CYP2B6, 87, 88, 91t
CYP2C19, 85, 87, 91t
CYP2C8, 90t
CYP2C9, 91t, 154
CYP2D6, 83, 87, 144
CYP2E1, 83, 90, 91, 91t
CYP3A4, 83, 87, 89–90, 90t, 164
CYP450, 83, 86, 89–91, 97, 142, 154, 163
cytochrome P450 (CYP450) enzymes, 83, 86, 89–91, 97, 142, 154, 163
cytokinesis, 27
cytoplasm, 17
cytosol, 17
cytotoxic drug action, 60
    antibacterial drugs, 131–132
    antiviral drugs, 132–133, 133t
    cancer pharmacology, 135
    and phases of cell cycle, 136f
    primary resistance, 137–138

secondary resistance, 138
working, 136–138

dabigatran, 106
dalteparin, 56
darunavir, 163, 164
deltoid site, for IM injection, 57, 58f
dendritic cells, 58
dephosphorylation, 26
dermis, 51
detectors/receptors, 4, 5
detoxification, 46
diamorphine, 94
diazepam, 47t, 91, 120
diffusion, 18, 20, 61
digoxin, 47t, 74, 77, 126t, 147–149
diphenhydramine, 121
distal convoluted loop, 102, 103f
disulfiram, 90
diuretics, 128
dobutamine, 92
dopamine, 119–120, 122
dopamine agonists, 120
dopamine antagonists, 122, 152
dorsogluteal site, for IM injection, 57, 58f
doxorubicin, 128
doxycycline, 33
drug absorption, 29
    food on, 40
    mechanisms of, 32
drug action, principles of, 113–114, 114t
    agonist, 119–120, 124t, 124f
    allosteric modulator, 125
    antagonists, 122–124, 124t, 124f
    carrier protons as target sites, 127–129
    cell receptors, 116–119
    cytotoxic drug action, 131–135
    enzyme inhibition as target site, 129–131, 129f
    full agonists, 120
    inverse agonists, 121–122
    and names, 3t
    partial agonists, 120–121
    selectivity, 125–126, 126t
    side effects and adverse drug responses, 114–116
    specificity, 126
drug administration
    bioavailability, 46–48, 47t
    buccal and sublingual routes, 48–50, 49f
    enteral route of, 30–38
    first-pass metabolism, 45–46, 46f
    intra-arterial, 60–62
    parenteral routes of, 55–60
    routes of, 30
    topical and transdermal administration, 50–55
drug clearance, 105–107

drug distribution, 73f
    body-related factors, 77–78
    definition of, 63–64
    drug-related factors, 76–77
    factors affecting, 76–78
    VoD. *See* volume of distribution (VoD) of drug
drug–drug interactions, 40
drug excretion
    breast milk, 110
    drug clearance, 105–107
    exhaled air, 109
    hepatobiliary system, 109
    *See also* kidneys
drug–food interactions, 40–41
drug metabolism, 42
    concepts and principles of, 79–82
    CYP450 enzyme induction and enzyme inhibition, 89–91
    entero-hepatic recycling, 91, 91f
    enzyme, in gut, 42, 46
    factors affecting
        age, 86
        disease, 88
        environmental factors, 88
        ethnicity, 87
        gender, 87
        genetic factors, 84–86
        pregnancy, 87
    final drug metabolism, 80
    first-pass metabolism, 80
    half-life of drug, 92–95, 94f
    hepatic enzymes, 82–84
    induction, 163
    liver, anatomy and physiology of, 80–82, 80f, 81f
    mechanisms, 83
    metaboliser types, 86f
    phases of, 79–82, 82f, 83
    phenotypical changes in CYP metabolism, 85t
    prodrugs, 95–97
    therapeutic window and therapeutic index, 97–98
drug nomenclature, 2
drugs
    administered dose of, 66
    affecting action of cytochrome P450 enzymes, 90–91t
    dissolution of, 42
    and food, levels of absorption in, 41t
    half-life of, 92–95
    highly polar and low lipophilicity, 64
    low polarity and high lipophilicity, 64
    moderately polar/lipophilicity, 64
    physical and chemical properties of, 43–44
    polarity of, 38–39
    properties of common, 64t

and receptors, 119
selectivity, 97
*See also specific entries*

eczema, 52
efavirenz, 133t
effectors, 4, 5
efficacy, 9, 120
elbasvir, 133t
electrolytes, 12, 13t
electroporation, 54
elements, 7, 7t
emollients, 52
emtricitabine (FTC), 163
enalapril, 96, 129
endocrine signalling, 25
endocytosis, 18, 23
endogenous insulin, 55
endoplasmic reticulum (ER), 17
enfuvirtide, 133t
enoxaparin, 56
enterohepatic recirculation, 37
entero-hepatic recycling, 91, 91f, 109
enzyme-catalysed reaction, products of, 15f
enzyme inhibition, 89
    ACE inhibitors, 129–130
    anticholinesterases, 131
    aspirin and inhibition of
        cyclo-oxygenase, 130
    enzyme catalysis vs, 129f
    monoamine oxidase inhibitors, 130–131
    as target site of drug action, 129–131
enzyme-linked receptors, 118t
enzymes, 9, 15–16
epidermis, 51
ER (extended release), 43
erythromycin, 53
ethanol, 109
excretion, 24, 101, 102
exhaled air, 109
exocytosis, 18, 23
external respiration, 61
extracellular fluid (ECF), 10, 12

fat/water ratio, 77
felodipine, 42
fentanyl, 54
filtration, 22
final drug metabolism, 80
first-pass metabolism, 36, 38, 45–46, 46f, 80
flucloxacillin, 40
flumazenil, 125
fluoride (F), 7t
5-fluorouracil, 137
fluoxetine, 47t
flu vaccine, 58
fosamprenavir, 96
fosfomycin, 160

full agonists, 120
furosemide, 147–148

GABA (gamma-aminobutyric acid)
    receptors, 138
gastrin, 34–35
gastrointestinal epithelium, 32, 55
gastrointestinal tract (GIT), 30, 31f
    anatomical regions, 30
    bacteria in, 45
    barriers, 32
    changes to pH within, 39
    colon, 44–45
    functional integrity of, 41
    intestine, 35–38, 45
    major layers of, 31, 31f
    stomach, 33–35, 34f
generic name, 2
gentamicin, 38, 107
glomerular filtration, 104
glomerular filtration rate (GFR), 104
glomerulonephritis, 75
glomerulus, 102
glyceryl trinitrate (GTN), 47, 48, 50
glycogen, 81
Golgi complex/Golgi apparatus, 18
G protein-coupled receptors, 118t
grazoprevir (Zepatier), 133t
gut motility, 38, 39f
    age-related reduction in, 42
    reduction in, 42
gut transit time, 38

$H_1$-antihistamines, 121
half-life of drug, 92–95, 94f, 95t
HCl, 34
hemin, 160
heparin, 56
hepatic enzymes, 82–84
hepatitis A, 132
hepatitis C, 133t
herbal supplements and prescribed
    medications (case study), 141–143
herpes zoster (shingles) viral
    infections, 133t
histamine antagonists, 121
homeostasis, 3–4
homeostatic control
    of blood pressure, 5–6
    of respiration, 5
human herpes simplex virus (HSV), 133t
human immunodeficiency virus (HIV), 133t
humectants, 52
hydrogen, 9–10
hydrogen ions, 10
hydrolysis, 83
hydromorphone, 106
hydromorphone-3-glucuronide, 106

hydrophilic/hydrophobic (water soluble drugs), 18, 63, 64t, 68, 77
hypernatraemia, 13
hypertension, 123
hypertensive emergencies, 92
hyperthyroidism, 88
hypertonic solution, 21
hypoalbuminemia, 75
hypodermis, 51
hypokalaemia, 148
hyponatraemia, 13
hypotonic solution, 21

ibuprofen, 72, 126t, 147–148
ileum, 35, 41, 44
influenza A and B, 133t
inhalation, 60–62, 61f
injection, recommended sites for, 56, 56f, 58f
inner renal medulla, 101
insulin, 39, 55
International Nonproprietary Names (INN), 2
interphase, cell cycle, 27
interstitial fluid (IF), 12
intestinal flora, 36
intestine, 35–38
intra-arterial drug administration, 60–62
intracellular fluid (ICF), 10
intracellular steroid, 118t
intramuscular (IM) administration, 55, 57–58
intravenous (IV) drug administration, 55, 59–60
    advantages, 59
    disadvantages, 60
inverse agonists, 121–122
iodine (I), 7t
ion, 10
ionic compounds, 8
ionised (polar) substances, 104
iontophoresis, 54
iron (Fe), 7t
ischaemic cardiomyopathy, 141
isocarboxazid, 130
isoprenaline, 126
isosorbide mononitrate, 47
isotonic solution, 21

jejunum and ileum, pathology affecting, 41

keratinocytes, 51
kidneys
    anatomy of, 101–108, 102f
    drug clearance, 105–107
    glomerular filtration, 104
    tubular reabsorption, 104
    tubular secretion, 104–105

lactase, 16
Langerhans cells, 51
laxatives, 29
lethal dose (LD), 98
levodopa, 40, 71
ligand, 24, 27, 116, 119
ligand-gated ion channels, 117t
lipases, 15–16
lipohypertrophy, 55–56
lipophilic (lipid soluble drugs), 33, 63, 64t, 68, 77, 82
lipoproteins, 72
lisdexamfetamine, 96
lisinopril, 97, 129
lithium, 47t, 73, 105, 107
lithium therapy (case studies), 149–151, 161–162
liver, anatomy and physiology of, 80–82, 80f, 81f
loading dose (LD), 68
local anaesthetics, 9
loperamide, 71–72
lorazepam, 91
low-dose aspirin, for antiplatelet therapy, 145–146
lymphatic system, 36
lymph nodes, 58
lysosomes, 18

major calyx, 101
malabsorption syndrome, 41
maltase, 16
manganese (Mn), 7t
Medicines and Healthcare products Regulatory Agency (MHRA), 115
medulla oblongata, 5
mefenamic acid, 106
melanocytes, 51
Merkel cells, 51
metabolic absorption, 23
metabolism, 82
metabolite, 83
metformin, 106, 107
methadone, 163–164
methotrexate, 106
methylphenidate patch, 54
metoclopramide, 38, 40, 151–153
microneedles, 54
microtubules, 18
microvilli, 18, 36
midazolam, 50, 139
milrinone, 93
minor calyx, 101
mitochondria, 17
mitosis, 24
mitotic (M) phase, 27
mivacurium, 84
molecular size, of drug molecule, 77
molecules, 6
    versus compounds, 8
molybdenum (Mo), 7t

6-monoacetylmorphine (6-MAM), 94
monoamine oxidase (MAO) enzyme, 130–131
morphine, 106, 139
morphine-6-glucuronide, 76, 93, 106
morphine sulphate, 46, 80, 97, 115, 139
movement, 23
MR (modified release), 43
mucosa, 31, 61
mucus, 32, 35
mu (μ) receptors, 115
mu–opioid receptors, 125, 139
muscarinic receptor, 123f
muscularis externa, 31
myasthenia gravis, 131

naloxone, 93, 121, 122, 125, 143–144
narrow therapeutic index drugs (NTIDs), 74
narrow therapeutic range, 157
National Institute for Health and Care Excellence (NICE), 53
neostigmine bromide, 131
nephron loop (loop of Henle), 102, 103f
nephrons, 102
nephrotic syndrome, 75
neurotransmitter, 119, 127
nicotinic receptor, 123f
nifedipine, 47t
nitrofurantoin, 106, 158, 160
nitroglycerin, 48
nitroprusside, 92
nociceptors, 130
non-competitive (irreversible) antagonists, 123
non-steroidal anti-inflammatory drugs (NSAIDs), 32, 106, 107, 126t, 130, 146
noradrenaline, 124
norepinephrine, 127
nuclear hormone receptors, 118t
nucleus, 16

oesophagus, 33
olanzapine, 122
omeprazole, 40, 126
opioid, 54
oral transmucosal, 48–50
oseltamivir, 96, 133t
osmoreceptors, 13
osmosis, 12, 20–21
osmotic pressure, 21
outer renal cortex, 101
oxidation, 83

paclitaxel, 128
pancreas, 37
paracrine signalling, 25
parenteral routes of drug administration, 55–60
 intramuscular administration, 55, 57–58
 intravenous route, 55, 59–60
 subcutaneous injection, 55–57
partial agonists, 120–121
pepsins, 35
perfusion, 48
 in drug distribution, 76
P-glycoprotein (P-gp) inhibitors, 70, 72, 128, 129
pH, 3, 9–10, 76
pH scale, 10f, 11f
pharmacodynamics, 2
 factors affecting, 138–140
  age, 138–139
  receptor activation and responsivity, 139–140
 principles of, 113–140
 See also drug action, principles of; cytotoxic drug action
pharmacogenetics, 84
pharmacokinetics, 2
 interactions (case study), 154–158
pharmacology, 1
phenelzine, 130
phenobarbitone, 91
phenoxybenzamine, 123–124
phenytoin, 42, 84
pheochromocytoma, 123
phosphate, 14
phosphodiesterase enzymes, 157
phospholipids, 14, 18, 19f
phosphoramide mustard, 97
phosphorylation cascade, 26
pinocytosis, 23
plasma, 12
plasma membrane, 18–19, 19f
plasma protein binding, 72–75
 factors affecting, 73–75
  age, 74–75
  competition for binding sites, 74
  disease, 75
  ethnicity, 75
  saturation of sites, 74
polarity of drug, 38–39
pons varolii, 5
porphyrins, 159
potassium, 13, 148
potency, 120
prednisolone, 142
prednisone, 96
pre-systemic metabolism. See first-pass metabolism
primary resistance, 137–138
procyclidine, 152
prodrugs, 47
pro-drugs, 84, 95–97
prokinetic agents, 40
propofol, 76, 77
propranolol, 46, 115, 126t

prostaglandins, 130, 146
protein–drug complex, 72
protein factories, 17
protein kinases, 26–27
proton pump inhibitors (PPIs), 10, 39, 127
proximal convoluted tubule, 102, 103f
pulmonary excretion, 109
pyridostigmine bromide, 131

quadrate lobe, 80
quetiapine, 122
quinidine, 106

receptor down-regulation, 139
receptors, 116–117, 117–118t
rectum, 45
rectus femoris, 58f
reduction reactions, 83
renal clearance, 104, 108
renal corpuscle, 102
renal papilla, 101
renal pyramids, 101
renal tubule, 102, 103f
renin-angiotensin-aldosterone pathway, 5
reproduction, 24
respiration, 24
  homeostatic control of, 5
respiratory acidosis, 9
respiratory control centres, 5
respiratory depression, 143
respiratory/metabolic disorders, 9
ribosomes, 17
rifampicin, 109
risperidone, 122
Ro15-4513, 121–122

salbutamol, 62, 126
saliva, 110
secondary resistance, 138
second messengers, 27
secretion, 24, 34–35
selectivity, of drug, 125–126, 126t
selegiline, 130
selenium (Se), 7t
semi-permeable membrane, 18, 21f
serosa, 31
serotonin, 127, 146
side effects and adverse drug
  responses, 114–116
signal transduction pathways model, 26f
sildenafil (Viagra), 126
simvastatin, 90
skeletal muscle, 57, 57f
skin, 50–51
  dermis, 51
  epidermis, 51
  hypodermis, 51
  layers of, 50f

small intestine, 35–38, 37f, 42
smoking cessation, 154–158
sodium, 7, 13, 22
sodium bicarbonate, 104
sodium thiopental, 93
solute concentration, in body
  compartments, 21
solutes, 12
solvent, 60
sonophoresis, 54
specificity, 126
SR (sustained release), 43
SSRIs (selective serotonin re-uptake
  inhibitors), 85, 122, 146
steroids, 32
St John's Wort, 89, 142
stomach, 33–35, 34f
stratum corneum, 53
subcutaneous (SC) administration, 55–57
subcutaneous layer. *See* hypodermis
sublingual administration, of drug, 48
submucosa, 31
suboptimal immunosuppression, 142
substrate, 15
sub-therapeutic, 89
succinylcholine, 84
sulfasalazine, 43
sulfonamide, 74, 75
synapse, 25
synaptic cleft, 118
synaptic transmission, 118f
systemic therapies, 135

tenofovir alafenamide (TAF), 163
tetracycline, 40
theophylline, 154–158
therapeutic drug monitoring (TDM),
  155, 157
therapeutic index (TI), 74, 98
therapeutic ratio. *See* therapeutic index (TI)
therapeutic window, 48, 98
thiopurine methyltransferase (TPMT)
  genotype, 85
thromboxane, 130
tinzaparin, 56
tolerance, 139
topical and transdermal drugs, 50–55
toxic dose (TD), 98
toxicity, 32
trace elements, 7
trademark name, 2
tramadol, 121
transdermal medication, 52, 52f, 53–55
transduction pathways, 26–27
trimethoprim, 106
trimethoprim-sulfamethoxazole, 160
trypsin, 16
tubular reabsorption, 104

tubular secretion, 104–105
tubulin, 18
type 1 diabetes, 55

urinary tract infections (UTIs), treating, 107

vacuole (vesicles), 18
valacyclovir, 96
valdecoxib, 130
vancomycin, 78, 106
varicella (chickenpox), 133t
vastus lateralis, 58f
vecuronium, 123
ventrogluteal site, for IM injection, 57, 58f
verapamil, 90, 128
villi, 36
vinblastine, 128
volume of distribution (VoD) of
    drug, 64–75
  blood–brain barrier (BBB), 69–72
  body-related factors and individual's
    physiology, 69
  calculating, 65, 67
  compartment model of, 65f
  equation, 66–67
  factors influencing, 68–75
  impact, 68
  loading dose (LD), 68
  plasma protein binding, 72–75

warfarin, 72–73, 153–154
water, 10–12, 20–21
withdrawal jumping, 121
World Health Organization (WHO), on side
  effect, 114

xanthopsia, 148

zidovudine, 133t
zinc (Zn), 7t